Table of Contents

Prologue

The Yiddish word *beshert* translates as some combination of "destiny" and "fate." It's been a theme running through Jay Levy's life, as this book documents. To understand it, consider the story of how Jay and I met.

We share an alma mater, Wesleyan University, though we graduated 30 years apart (1960 and 1990). Our paths never crossed – and seemed destined not to. He was a scientist based in San Francisco and I was a writer based in the Washington, D.C., area. But on Bastille Day in 2018, we were both at a social event in Northern California. The MC mentioned the presence of someone named "Jay Levy." I had not heard that name since seeing it in an article about him in a Wesleyan publication 30 years earlier. The fact that I saw the article, and remembered it decades later, could be chalked up to *beshert.*

I wondered if this could be the same person. I approached him and asked, "Did you go to Wesleyan?" "Yes!" he beamed. He was thrilled to meet someone else who had also spent four years in Middletown, Connecticut. He invited me to lunch soon thereafter and over time we became friends. We often talked about the very active life he had lived – including his time at Wesleyan, where we both served on the school's Board of Trustees (his term began immediately after my term as a student trustee ended).

It was also *beshert* that a graduate of Jay's beloved Wesleyan would also become his biographer. This book got its start as an offhand comment I made to Jay one afternoon in 2021, as we took a walk in Mountain Lake Park near his home in San Francisco's Richmond District. After hearing his many stories, I said he should write a book about his life. He was intrigued by the idea, but he eventually proposed to me that *I* should write a book about him. I was happy to do so and what you're reading is the product of that conversation.

The material for this book has largely come from interviews I conducted with Jay over a 15-month period. Sitting in the lower-level study of his San Francisco home, which is filled with mementoes from the many trips taken by he and his wife, Sharon, he would methodically walk me through different periods (and episodes) of his life – from childhood through to the present day – with remarkable clarity.

What I found during these interviews, and which I've tried to show in the pages that follow, is someone who has always been a natural extrovert and possessed with innate curiosity about people and places throughout the world. The byproducts of those traits are a diverse collection of friends and experiences spanning several decades, with deep personal connections to people and cultures representing disparate countries, including France, Greece, Indonesia, and Israel.

In the 1980s, Jay's curiosity, his global experiences, and his determination to solve medical mysteries, converged. The result was his pathbreaking insights into the fundamentals of HIV/AIDS – insights that were later cited as pivotal by a winner of the Nobel Prize, Luc Montagnier.

This book documents Jay's countless *beshert* moments throughout his life. (One of them, involving a classified ad in the *Washington Post*, led him to meet his wife, Sharon.) He has enabled these *beshert* moments through his travels, his socializing, and his curiosity. While in medical school, he learned of a philosopher in England who said that energy expended in one direction will come back in another direction. This became a guiding principle throughout Jay's life and he's been reminded of it again and again.

Consistent with the *beshert* theme, one of Jay's favorite books is *The Celestine Prophecy*. Published in 1993, it's a fictional account of one man's spiritual journey. A key idea in the book is that nothing happens by chance and seemingly random events need to be understood as a potential guide to the future – a principle he embraced two decades earlier when living in San Francisco. "The book has strongly influenced my decision making ever since I read it," says Jay. "Explore the details and nature of your experiences," he counsels. "There may be a message there. It's often helped me validate my decision-making."

Jay turned 87 during the writing of this book and he still had a crystal-clear recollection of events stretching back to his childhood. He and Sharon kept up an active travel schedule and he was still striving to cultivate new skills. In the spring of 2025, he began taking ukelele lessons – having first started playing the instrument in youth while working as a summer camp counselor.

My interviews with Jay revealed the multiple dimensions of his life. There's been the trailblazing research, of course, which rests on a foundation of resilience, focus, and curiosity that have enabled him to thrive. But there's also been teaching and mentoring outside the classroom, an active social life, and exotic travel. The result has been a life well lived.

To Dick Miller,

A great man whose commitment to friendship and fellowship made this book possible – and so much else

Chapter 1

Growing Up

In 1898, a 26-year-old Belarusian Jew named Reuben Lapidus arrived on Ellis Island, just below the southern tip of Manhattan. It was the destination for millions of immigrants to the United States, from throughout the world. He was fleeing the antisemitic pogroms that periodically threatened his small village outside Minsk, in modern-day Belarus.

Reuben told the immigration officials his family name was "Levy," figuring this would help him find a Jewish community, in which to live. ("Levy" was a much more common Jewish surname than "Lapidus.") He was told he could find one in an unlikely destination: Delaware. More specifically, Wilmington, the small state's largest city, with a population of about 60,000 at the time.

Reuben took a small steamer down the Delaware River to Wilmington. There he lived on the poor side of the river and set up a shoe repair shop on Front Street – his father had been a shoemaker – in the city's Jewish neighborhood. He lived in the rear of the store that he rented.

Reuben was already married when he came to the United States. His wife, Leah, had stayed behind in Belarus to care for their two young children, Abraham and Florence. Reuben returned to the old country in 1904 and stayed until 1905, because of the Russo-Japanese war. He traveled back to Wilmington alone, because there wasn't enough money for anyone else. Ruben returned to Delaware almost every year, and the Levy family grew in size.

The plan was for Leah and the children to join Reuben in Wilmington, and the family arrived throughout the 1890s and 1900s. In 1907, Reuben tried to bring two of the children, but they had a viral eye disease known as trachoma and he had to return to Belarus with them and Leah. Once the trachoma was successfully treated, the children returned to Wilmington, with Leah. By 1911, the entire family, which featured seven children, was living in Philadelphia, where they were met by a cousin with the family name Shapiro.

The fifth child, Charles, had been born in Belarus in 1905. When he was six, he lived in Wilmington with his father and mother in a room behind the shoe store. The family also had a shoe store in Philadelphia, which had some extra rooms. Charles also lived there with four other children for several years.

Charles was an academic standout and graduated from Wilmington High School in just two years. He then enrolled at the University of Delaware, where he co-founded a Jewish fraternity and made lifelong friends. One of them, Philip Blank, had a younger sister named Ruth. She and Charles met when she was just 16 and he was 26. They quickly became a couple and married five years later, in Newark, New Jersey.

Charles completed his studies at the University of Delaware in three years and then went to medical school in Philadelphia, at Thomas Jefferson University. He graduated in three years, which meant that at the tender age of just 23 he was already seeing patients. Ruth and Charles eventually bought a house for $18,000 in a new suburban community called Carrcroft, about five miles north of downtown Wilmington, at 206 Rowland Park Boulevard.

Charles had a fraternity brother, Hyman Albert Yanowitz – he changed his last name to "Young" and went by "Hy" – who became a close friend and married Ruth's older sister, Ann. Hy graduated from the University of

Pennsylvania law school and set up his practice in Wilmington. In 1951, he became the attorney general for the state of Delaware, which made him one of a small number of American Jews at the time to have been a statewide elected official.

On November 21, 1938, Ruth gave birth to twins, Stuart and Jay, in Wilmington General Hospital. Both weighed more than eight pounds. Stuart was born first. Jay arrived 20 minutes later – in a hallway of the hospital, while Ruth was being wheeled to the recovery room to wait for the placenta. Given the state of medical technology at the time, Ruth and Charles never knew she was pregnant with twins.

Jay was named in memory of Ruth's uncle, who had recently died in a car accident, while Stuart was named in memory of Ruth's late father, Samuel. (A tradition among American Jews is for babies to sometimes be given a first name that starts with the same letter as the person being honored.) Jay and Stuart also received a Hebrew name. Stuart's was Casir and Jay's was Yehuda. They were identical twins, born from one placenta. Stuart had one distinguishing feature at birth: a small bump on his forehead. The family joke was that the bump stemmed from Jay's push to have Stuart exit the birth canal before him.

The birth order led Charles to refer to Stuart and Jay as "number one" son and "number two" son throughout their lives. (The labels were likely inspired by Charlie Chan TV shows, which Jay's father enjoyed.) Because Stuart was born first, Charles concluded he would be the more responsible son. As a result, recalls Jay, "when left to a decision between my brother and me, Stuart always was chosen and was therefore considered most dependable. That did not bother me since it freed me up to be a little more adventuresome."

Soon after Jay and Stuart were born, their parents hired a full-time housekeeper and cook, Grace, and a full-time maid, Nancy. (Grace, a strict disciplinarian, occupied one of the home's four bedrooms, while Nancy, a descendant of slaves, had a bed in the home's basement.) They were needed to help with the two boys, as well as a sister, Ellen, who was born in 1941. Charles – a general practitioner, who later had a specialty in cardiology and diabetes – was often gone in the evening, as he typically made house calls to patients (as many doctors did at the time). Whenever the boys would ask where he was, their mother would reply, "out saving lives." And Charles once rescued a woman who was choking by opening her windpipe with a knife.

Ruth would sometimes accompany Charles on house calls. They were often paid via barter – in exchange for medical services, they might be given a meal or sometimes a live chicken. Charles made house calls for many years and only stopped after doctors started being robbed for the drugs they carried.

A lesson in the value of medicine came when Jay was just 18 months old and diagnosed with osteomyelitis. This bone infection in his left foot left him hospitalized for several months and the infection was treated by removing some of the infected bone. Jay was given what was a new drug at the time – sulfur. The drug had been brought home from World War II by a friend of Charles (and fellow doctor), Joseph Barsky. "Uncle Joe" was also the godfather to Jay and Stuart.

The sulfur cured Jay of what could have been a debilitating – and even deadly – condition. Nevertheless, he had to wear a special boot on his left foot into his teenage years, and the boot subjected him to teasing from his peers. "My dad told Stuart to look after me, and he always stayed protective of me until I was married," recalls Jay.

One legacy of the infection is a smaller left foot (the osteomyelitis curbed its growth), with a shrunken fourth toe – the one next to his little toe. The other legacy is Jay's career. "When I was old enough to understand osteomyelitis and how I was cured by sulfur, it sparked an interest in medicine," recalls Jay. "I wanted others to benefit from medicine, just as I had. Interestingly, my parents never pushed me or Stuart or Ellen to become doctors." It was an early example of the resilience and determination that would become hallmarks of Jay's life.

World War II

The earliest years of Jay's childhood coincided with World War II. One of his few memories – the war ended when Jay was 6 – was his dad creating a mock infirmary in the basement of the family home. "I remember peeking into the basement when I was 4 or 5 and seeing several cots with white sheets," recalls Jay. "They were filled with people pretending to be wounded, with other people pretending to care for them. And there were several nights when we would turn off all the lights because we thought our neighborhood could be bombed if its location was identified."

Jay and Stuart, along with their dad, also planted what was known as a "victory garden," where they tended to tomatoes, corn, and carrots. The US government encouraged people to start these gardens, as a way to free up agricultural produce for soldiers. And the Levy family was far from alone in making this patriotic gesture. By 1944, 18.5 million people had planted such gardens, and they were estimated to generate 40 percent of the nation's fresh vegetables.

Jay recalls while in the garden one day, he came across a praying mantis, which seemed exotic to him. "My dad said not to kill it, because they consumed the mosquitos." Following the war's end, the Levy victory garden evolved into a landscaped garden after a failed attempt at a pond – planted by the boys and Ellen, with wild dogwoods and tulip poplar trees.

In April 1945, FDR died. Jay was in the car with his mother when she learned of the death, from the radio. She cried, "We lost a very great and important man."

Judaism

Germany made the eradication of Jews from Europe a central plank of its war effort, but the Levy children were young at the time and religion played only a small role in their lives. "It was not emphasized" recalls Jay. "There was no antisemitism evident to us at that age in Wilmington."

When Jay and Stuart were about 6 years old, they started going to Hebrew school twice a week. And two years before the boys' bar mitzvahs, which was held at their Conservative synagogue, Beth Shalom, they would go three times per week. But for Jay, a big draw of Hebrew school was the opportunity to visit a classic soda fountain, Gasser's, afterwards. (The bus to the Levy home picked up the riders just outside the store's front door.)

Out of respect for their Russian grandparents, the family kept kosher at home, and were observant of the High Holidays, but not other holidays, such as *sukkot.* During the High Holidays, Jay's parents would stay with a relative, often Uncle Abe, so they could walk to Beth Shalom. Jay's paternal grandparents, Reuben and Leah, were more observant – Reuben attended an Orthodox synagogue and spent much of his time each day praying. "He would take a break and put his hands on my head," recalls Jay, "I felt as if he was absolving me of all my sins." (Charles had been brought up in an Orthodox synagogue, but once he had settled in Carrcroft and after his parents died, he followed his friends and relatives in joining Beth Shalom.)

Each Yom Kippur, relatives would come to the Ruben and Leah's home for an annual tradition known as *slot kapparot.* It involved swinging a live chicken by its legs, above one's head, seven times, while repeating prayers. This activity was supposed to pass your sins to the chicken, which was then cooked and eaten by the family at the end of the holiday. "I hoped that the sins were killed by cooking them," recalls Jay.

When Reuben was near death, he wrote a letter that was addressed to his children and urged them to maintain their bonds to Judaism.

> I beg of you, beloved children, to always conduct yourselves as Jews, in practice, and primarily in your homes; teach your children to be proper Jews, true to the Jewish nation, dedicated to the land; implant in them all that is Jewish, so that they will never forget they are Jews; teach your children to respect the Jewish national the Jewish religion; help out, to the best of your capabilities, Jewish institutions; do not skimp from giving money for Zion and Jerusalem.

Everyday life

As a brutal war was being fought throughout the world, the Levy family lived comfortably, with a four-bedroom house and two full-time staff. Charles, who also bought a modest home in Wilmington for his parents, Reuben and Leah, drove a Cadillac and Ruth a Chevrolet. They would take trips often to Florida for the winter – typically without Jay, Stuart, and Ellen. Even so, recalls Jay, "being alone without parents led to strong bonding between me, Stuart, and Ellen." When the parents returned, the three kids would typically put on a short show with costumes and singing, and their dog Connie as the star.

One unfortunate family episode was a byproduct of some mischief imagined by Jay and Stuart. Around the age of 5 or 6, they were playing in their bedroom one evening with an article of clothing, to see what it would feel like against their skin if it was warmed up by an electric heater. The clothing caught fire, so they threw it in their trash can. But the flame wasn't fully extinguished. It eventually ignited and burned the entire bedroom. Fire trucks came and the boys had to exit the house via a ladder. The neighbors, the Ploeners, were alerted and came to help. Charles and Ruth thought the fire stemmed from an electrical defect and had the home's electrical wiring evaluated. The boys didn't reveal what actually happened for another 10 years, during a regular family gathering in their parents' bedroom. "They were relieved to hear the truth," recalls Jay, "and nothing more was ever said about it."

Sometime later, Jay's mischievous side emerged again – he decided to run away from home one afternoon. But it only amounted to hiding behind bushes near the house. He was so close he tried to listen through the house's back windows to see if anyone noticed he was missing. Alas, he couldn't hear much and he returned to the house, meekly, for dinner. Grace, the housekeeper, showed no sympathy for Jay, and his mom was nonchalant, saying the little adventure should be ignored.

It was an otherwise happy childhood for Jay and Stuart. The two boys were free to roam in the neighborhood, riding their bicycles and looking for friends. They did the typical things boys of that age did, such as building a tree hut, which they would reach via a hidden ladder. And with other boys from different neighborhoods a few blocks away, they would have gang wars, which were more like low-level skirmishes. Homemade ice cream, made by the mother of one of the gang members, often followed their outings. But the environment wasn't entirely typical: one local eight-year-old boy taught them to play bridge.

Jay and Stuart were eager to follow some of their friends and start kindergarten at the age of 5. But Ruth didn't see the need for their formal education to begin, telling them, "You'll have plenty of time for school – go out and play."

Much of their play time was near a stream in the woods that was not far from the Levy family home and gardens. The boys would search for animals under rocks and nearby shrubs in the woods. Once, they found a rabbit nest, which led them to adopt the baby rabbits, who were fed milk with droppers. The rabbits were named "SPERJ," which came from the first letter of the first name of each member of the group. The "J" was for Joyce Tharp, who was the lone girl in the group. She didn't get any special treatment and was once tied to a tree by local boys.

Jay and Stuart had their first experience with bullying when they were 9 years old. They were returning from swimming in a river in Arden, a nearby town. They were often taunted by a group of bullies, who called them "Heckle and Jeckle," which were the names of two identical yellow-billed black birds in a popular newspaper comic strip at the time. To try to stop the taunting, Jay went fisticuffs with a much larger heavyset boy. While both boys ended up with a black eye, Jay recalls that "we had no more problems with bullies after that. We learned that at that age 'might' could be 'right.'"

The Ploener family lived next door to the Levy family. A basketball hoop near a large weeping willow separated the two houses. But the hoop was crushed by the weeping willow tree during Hurricane Hazel in 1954. The Duffy family also lived nearby, in a mansion. Their son, Richard, once took the Levy children to the cellar of their home, and showed them the passageway used for escaped slaves (the house was on the underground railroad). "That was our introduction to the presence of slavery in Delaware," recalls Jay.

Boys from the neighborhood as well as from school often played basketball together in the driveways of the Levys and Ploeners. Jay and Stuart enjoyed these gathering so much that their father voiced concern that they might fall behind in school. They convinced him not to worry.

This intervention by Charles was more the exception than the rule. "Dad played a limited role in our upbringing," recalls Jay. "He worked very hard at the office. Mother did most of the nurturing." The boys rarely played a sport with their dad, who was a strict disciplinarian, particularly when the boys misbehaved in the car or at the dinner table. He spanked Jay once after catching him in a lie.

Performing arts

Performing arts were important to the Levy family. They may have been influenced by the "concerts" they sometimes put on with their dad and their sister Ellen playing violin, and the boys playing the piano with four hands. By the time they were 10, they would sometimes take the bus to the town of Arden to see shows at the local theater, with performers such as Barbara Bel Geddes and her husband, Windsor Lewis. They also enjoyed singing together, with Charles often writing the words to familiar tunes that would be sung on birthdays or holidays. (The singalong tradition continues to this day in the extended Levy family.)

When Jay and Stuart were 9 or 10, their dad surprised them with a visit to Philadelphia (about 30 miles away). They went to an audition for a TV show called "The Children's Hour" and sang "It's a Big Wide

Wonderful World." But they forgot the performance would be televised and didn't dance or make hand gestures, which likely contributed to their not being selected to perform on the show.

When Jay and Stuart were in elementary school and junior high, one of the school's teachers, Mr. Hallowell, persuaded them to perform in a talent show that was modeled on a popular television show called "Your Hit Parade." They were popular with their fellow students and continued to perform all the way through high school. When they were in junior high, the uncle of one of their fellow students, the famous comedian Henny Youngman, said they were the best act he observed in the school's competition.

Jay also managed the production of a play while in high school and once had to step into one of the parts on short notice. He was coached by his friend Joyce Tharp, who would later become a professional actor. At one point in the production, he had a moment that called for him to step into the bathroom from the stage. His nervousness made him forget those lines. Soon thereafter, he once again exited the stage for the bathroom. He recovered his lines, which led the audience to laugh.

More exposure to the performing arts came when Charles surprised the family with a television, around 1954, though the screen was so small the family had to watch it through a magnifier. They enjoyed Milton Berle's weekly show, though the experience was often interrupted by Connie, the family dog, whose flatulence drove everyone out of the room. In 1956, Charles was on a cruise, serving as a traveling doctor for one of his patients. Berle was also on the cruise and Charles treated him for his heart problem. The episode was written about in a Wilmington newspaper and as a show of gratitude Berle sent Charles 100 neckties.

As the boys grew older, the family held annual football games, which took place on Thanksgiving and Christmas weekends. Motivated by natural competitive spirits of the Young boys and the Levy boys, the games were initially 2 vs. 2, but over time grew to include other family members, including girls, and had themes such as the "Crans" versus the "Berries" or the "Clauses" versus the "Santas." A trophy was created (the Youngs had more wins), but the twins developed strategies to gain an advantage, based on their youth and smaller size. The games were initially played in front of the Levy home or the Young home. It became an essential part of the holidays.

Elementary school

In September 1944, Jay and Stuart were enrolled at Harlan Elementary School, at 3601 Jefferson Street, a 15-minute car ride from Carrcroft. Their first-grade teacher was Mrs. Ruddert, who knew Jay's dad. She was a disciplinarian, as many teachers were at the time, and when Jay or Stuart misbehaved – they would occasionally talk when they were supposed to be quiet – she would pick them up by their hair and put them in the corner of the classroom. The two boys threatened to tell their father how they were being treated – but they never did. "We always wondered if we lost our hair later in life because of her," Jay recalled.

Throughout elementary school, Jay and Stuart enjoyed their classes – Jay was fascinated by dinosaurs in fourth grade. But they were competitive with each other and when they started at PS du Pont Junior High School in 1950, they were put in different classes. It was a *beshert* moment that their neighbor at the time, Cora Pickett, was the Dean at PS du Pont. She would drive them to school every morning and later helped arrange their placement in the best classes offered at the high school.

After each day of elementary school, Jay and Stuart traveled in a school bus back to their neighborhood. Their dog Connie – a boxer sometimes called "the Countess of Boxwood" – knew when the boys and Ellen would be arriving home on the school bus (probably from the position of the sun). She would meet them at the drop-off site, at the corner of Carr Road and Rowland Park Boulevard (Connie had been a gift from Jay's aunt – and his godmother – Frieda Barsky.) "That was a well appreciated late afternoon event," recalls Jay.

Summers

During the summers, Jay and Stuart attended traditional Jewish summer camps. The boys were shipped off to the first one, in Pennsylvania's Pocono Mountains, when they were just 7. But when Charles and Ruth came to visit, they found the boys covered in mud and sliding down a hill in the rain. They were withdrawn from the camp that afternoon.

During subsequent summers, the boys spent two months with their cousins, Stuart and Alan Young, at Camp Chickawah, in southern Maine. The days were filled with swimming (Jay learned to swim by being thrown into the camp's lake), boating, canoeing, sailing, wood rafting, and sometimes camping (with religious services every Friday). The lake where campers swam was infested with leeches, and the staff would nonchalantly pour salt over the leeches to displace them from the campers. This was not considered unusual and most of the parents knew this novel aspect of camp life.

Money was sometimes tight in the Levy household, and so at age 14 Jay and Stuart did not return to Camp Chickawah. Instead, they started holding down summer jobs closer to home. (These jobs had the benefit of being better paid.) This included working in an ice cream factory (owned by a friend of the family known as "Uncle Mike") and a leather outlet (which employed another friend of the family known as "Uncle Saul"). That outlet was in a poor part of Wilmington where many employees played the numbers game. The boys could see the gambling houses by looking down the street from the company's windows. They also recognized the raids handled by the police. Jay and Stuart amused themselves by writing numbers on the factory walls that were taken by the employees as signs of a number to bet on.

Jay also worked as a mailman in his neighborhood one Christmas season. Stuart filled in for him a few days a week, since the boys were identical twins. Several years later, Jay's dad shared this story with a retired postmaster general, who was not amused, pointing out that impersonating a mail carrier was a federal offense.

As noted above, the boys also worked at their Uncle Mike's ice cream factory in Wilmington. Jay was in a small room mimeographing "vanilla" on the side of cardboard boxes; Stuart helped to supervise the robot that delivered ice cream popsicles from the ceiling into boxes for transport to groceries. At times, the box robot jammed, which prompted a bell to ring and employees would rush to the floor to fill their pails with the unboxed ice cream popsicles. Jay always complained that he got the wrong end of the stick that time.

Jay also worked in the summer at the local horse track, breaking even at the end of the season with his salary covering his last-minute bets. He and Stuart were also hired by their dad to paint the white picket fence surrounding the family home, for which they were each paid 40 cents an hour.

The boys later worked as counselors at the all-boys Camp Powhatan, also in Maine, where they taught golf (they'd been given golf lessons as a bar mitzvah present by Herbert Steinberg, their father's good friend). They also composed some camp songs (set to the tune of classical music or popular tunes at the time) and helped direct some plays. The camp would hold dances with a nearby all-girls camp, and at one of those dances Jay had his first kiss.

One summer after finishing college, Jay worked as an inspector for the highway department. His job was to measure the size of the holes to be repaired by the road asphalt company. He thought he was doing a good job and was surprised when he would find a bottle of scotch in his locker, as a gift from the asphalt company. When one of the employees told him he didn't have to be so exact in measuring the size of the holes, he realized the reason for the scotch.

The summer jobs educated both boys on life "on the outside," which was precisely what their dad wanted. "My father wanted us to hold all of these different jobs, which typically involved a good bit of manual labor, so we would have a greater appreciation for the value of a college degree," recalls Jay. "It worked."

High school

Jay and Stuart attended P.S. du Pont High School, where they excelled academically, in an environment where the overwhelming share of their classmates were not planning to go to college. But it was still rigorous coursework – both Jay and Stuart took four years of Latin. "Our parents insisted we do well in Latin," and having their neighbor, Cora Pickett, assign them to classes with the best teachers was a great advantage.

His sophomore year, Jay took a class that involved reading the "great books" – such as those by Dickens, Hawthorne, and Tolstoy. This experience sparked his interest in American literature. He later wrote a paper on famous presidential speeches.

Jay also entered the state science fair a few times while in high school. One of his projects showed how herbs could be transformed into medicine. "It was a lot of work, but I loved doing it, and I think my dad liked it too," recalls Jay. The project won an "honorable mention" designation in the state fair, and for several weeks a poster that Jay made for the project hung in the window of a local pharmacy owned by a friend of the family.

Jay was sufficiently interested in science that during the fall of his sophomore year he wrote a letter to a professor of biochemistry at Johns Hopkins University, E.V. McCollum, asking about his research on rickets. He also requested a photo of McCollum, who complied with the request.

In high school, Jay and Stuart were on the track team. Even with his foot issue, Jay was very strong in the quarter mile and half mile and competed in the fabled Penn Relays in Philadelphia (with Stuart) against other high school runners. "I liked sports because they boosted my popularity and helped me develop friends," recalls Jay.

His real goal was to play football. Alas, his parents were adamantly opposed to him (and Stuart) joining the team. Instead, they became the football team's managers, which involved everything from keeping statistics to providing water for the players and helping the coaches. This activity kept them connected to the sport and the players, without incurring the inevitable injuries. They also earned a varsity letter, which meant more to them than the many other awards they received at graduation. "We learned that life can offer rewards in other ways," recalled Jay. "But you have to make the effort."

Both Jay and Stuart were the proverbial BMOCs (big men on campus), given their involvement in sports and the performing arts, as well as their strong academic standing. Their shared identity led to a remarkable moment: they ran against each other for student body president. They both held campaign strategy meetings in the family home – Jay in the dining room and Stuart in the living room. The parents didn't try to talk them out of it, recognizing that one of them would prevail. Jay's slogan was "Leave it to Levy" and his campaign posters featured a tree that had his goals printed on the tree's leaves.

Jay prevailed, as did his sister, Ellen, who was running to be president of the junior high. Jay congratulated her via the school's loudspeaker and he emphasized that there would be strong collaboration between the two schools. (She was later forced to serve as vice president, because it was thought a girl shouldn't serve as president.) The defeat did not seem to bother Stuart, who later won election as the school's student treasurer. And for Jay, the victory was special, having lost a re-election bid to the student council a few years earlier by 16 votes.

One of their friends, Phyllis Attick, was elected secretary. Her parents were close friends of Delaware's incumbent governor, Caleb Boggs, and they got him to speak at the student government inauguration party. Jay later recalled that this experience was the start of his appreciation for politics. In 1960, Jay wrote to Boggs and congratulated him on being elected to the US Senate. (A staff member wrote back to Jay and assured him that his letter to Boggs "will be brought to his attention.") Boggs was re-elected in 1966, but was defeated in 1972 by a young councilman from New Castle County named Joe Biden.

Amid their many achievements, Jay and Stuart were not above the occasional prank. Each April Fool's Day, they would swap class schedules. One year, Stuart was reprimanded and told to stay after school to meet with his English teacher. She demanded that he apologize for misbehaving in the class. He swore that he was not involved with this misbehavior. Jay later revealed that he and Stuart had switched classes that day, so he (Stuart) wasn't the truant.

On another April Fool's Day, the biology teacher was so upset by the prank that she warned them that they would probably think of switching classes in college, but they would be expelled if they did so. Jay and Stuart took that as a challenge,

Chapter 2

Wesleyan

It was early October 1956 – one month before Americans would vote for President. Dwight Eisenhower was running for reelection and had dispatched his running mate – Richard M. Nixon – to shore up support for the Republican ticket in New England. Nixon arrived at Bradley Field – the airport serving the Hartford, Connecticut metropolitan area – at 2:30 a.m. and was greeted by 50 young Republicans from nearby Wesleyan University. They welcomed him with posters, horns, and cowbells. Amid the throng of students was a bright-eyed and bespectacled Wesleyan freshman: Jay Levy.

Jay took a circuitous route to arriving at the small, all-male liberal arts college in central Connecticut. His first choice was Amherst, in neighboring Massachusetts; he was drawn to its small size (averaging about 200 students per class) and liberal arts education. With a robust high school resume marked by academic prowess, stellar extra-curricular activities, and a winning personality, Jay's acceptance seemed assured

Alas, college admissions were nearly as unpredictable in 1956 as they are today, and Amherst did not accept Jay. He was surprised, but he took solace in hearing a story that a student from his high school a few years earlier had gone to Amherst but floundered there, which may have led the admissions officers to question the value of anyone from the school.

Jay received better news from Wesleyan and immediately decided to accept the offer of admission – despite never having visited the campus. Around the same time, both Stuart and Jay were also accepted at Williams

College, in northwest Massachusetts, which was similar in size and reputation to Wesleyan. And, like Wesleyan, it was part of the "Little Three," along with Amherst. (Their cousin, Stuart Young, was already a student at Williams.) Jay and Stuart still had applications pending at Harvard, Yale, and Princeton – the larger, "Big Three" counterparts to the Little Three schools. Because other students in their high school class had applied to these schools and were waiting to hear from them, they both withdrew those applications.

One of Jay's earliest Wesleyan experiences was the late-night airport visit to see Richard Nixon. He had joined the College Republicans soon after arriving on campus, reflecting his extended family's political lineage. His uncle, Hy Young, had run successfully as a Republican for attorney general of Delaware. "I felt privileged to be in a group that was there," recalls Jay, "even though we had to wait about two hours for him to arrive. I later voted for him when he ran for President."

A few days after the event, the front page of Wesleyan's school newspaper, *The Argus,* featured a photo of Nixon and his wife Pat at the event, with a beaming (and bespectacled) Jay sandwiched between them.[1]

If there was any question whether Jay would be an outsized figure on campus, it was put to rest just 11 days later: Jay appeared in another photo on the front page of *The Argus* – this one connected to a school pep rally.[2]

It was an auspicious beginning, and Jay had quickly put his social skills to work, learning the names and backgrounds of his fellow students, while being impressed by the diversity and friendliness of his fellow students.

But it masked an unfortunate reality: Jay was unhappy in Middletown. Most Wesleyan freshmen lived in dorms, but he had been assigned to a house with 14 other students in a somewhat isolated part of the Wesleyan campus. (The house name was "So-est," as it was located in the southeast area of the campus.) He felt marginalized and not fully part of the Wesleyan community.

He was also surprised by the small number of Jews at the school – they only accounted for about 10 percent of his class, which reflected a quota in place at many of the country's top colleges and universities at the time. But one of the Jewish students happened to be his roommate, Mark Lischner. Jay recalls that on move-in day, his parents went to the Republican Party headquarters in Middletown and bought him large posters of Eisenhower and Nixon, which he hung above his bed. Later that evening, Lischner put up a poster of the Democratic Party's candidates for President and Vice President, Adlai Stevenson and Estes Kefauver, respectively. "Mark and I became good friends, but our friendship didn't include politics," recalls Jay. "But having Mark as a roommate was an early *beshert* moment."

Jay visited Stuart at Williams one weekend, and while there he met students who were the sons of famous people, such as Bing Crosby and the president of General Motors. "I was left feeling that Wesleyan was not as popular as Williams," says Jay.

When Jay came home for Thanksgiving, he brought all his clothes with him and told his parents he was unhappy at Wesleyan and didn't want to return. His parents were alarmed, but his father insisted he return, which Jay did, reluctantly, riding back with another Wesleyan student from Wilmington.

A close bond with Lischner helped buoy Jay's spirits. Lischner grew up in Hartford, which was only about 20 minutes by car from Wesleyan, and his parents took him and Jay to dinner nearly every weekend at a restaurant called the Seafood Peddler. "That was very special for me," recalls Jay, "and made me feel at home."

At the start of the second semester, Jay was transferred from So-Est to a freshman dorm, Butterfield, that had just opened. It was close to the main library and the science center and it offered a sense of community with other freshmen that was lacking at So-Est. "I was extremely happy there," recalls Jay. "It was exactly the atmosphere I was looking for."

Newly energized, Jay put his organizational talents to work. He successfully petitioned Wesleyan's athletic department to start a freshman golf team (all other sports had a dedicated freshman team). And he served as a cheerleader for the football team. He also drew on his performing experience with Stuart and organized a singing group that was composed of ten of his fellow freshmen. He held tryouts for the group, which he called the Dixchords. Those selected were Jack Fowler, Charles Jacobs, James Corrodi, Phil Young, Jan Hogendorn, Steve Jones, Mark Lischner, James Dingfelder, and Gil Seeley.[3] The group performed at fraternity parties and other Wesleyan events.

By the end of freshman year, Jay recalls "feeling great" about Wesleyan. That summer, he and Stuart returned to Camp Powhatan in Maine as camp counselors and taught golf. Their time together that summer may have provided some inspiration for a remarkable prank they pulled off early in the second semester of their sophomore year: they switched schools for a week. Jay assumed the identity of Stuart at Williams, and Stuart did the same as Jay at Wesleyan. They each told six of their on-campus friends, and a few school officials knew, but no one else. The campus friends were called "relay men" and their job was to never leave one of the twins alone. That way some information about students they met could be whispered and used.

The prank was later revealed on the front page of Wesleyan's school newspaper, *The Argus,* and in the *Hartford Courant.* The *Argus* article included a photo of the twins, under the headline:

"Jay Returns To Wesleyan, Stu To Williams; Twins Reveal Complete Identity Hoax Story."

The details on a novel experiment in intercollegiate living were revealed to the Argus recently in an interview with Jay and Stuart Levy. Jay is a sophomore at Wesleyan, and his twin brother, Stuart is in the same class at Williams. Last week, with the permission of the deans,(obtained last year) they exchanged places at their respective schools.

On the weekend of February 8 Jay arrived in Williamstown for the [Williams] Winter Carnival. On Sunday Stuart returned to Middletown in Jay's place while Jay settled down in his "new" room in the sophomore dorms to prepare for his future experiences.

Six boys on each campus, including Jay's roommate, Mark Lischner, were informed of the plan so they, acting as relaymen, could take each twin to class and help him to know his brother's friends. Handbooks as well as yearbooks were exchanged so that the pictures inside could aid the boys in identifying other classmates.

The week before the hoax, Jay and Stuart made maps of their respective classrooms, outlined events for each day, and drew up descriptions of various people on campus whom they might run into. It was understood that they were to attend all classes and extra-curricular activities and interview as many faculty members as possible. Stuart even had to take a music exam for Jay which he is certain he flunked. Fortunately, with the deans in on the plan, this matter can be remedied.

The boys noted as many of their own idiosyncrasies as they could remember—food tastes, particular reactions to certain people, even times to go to meals and take showers. They kept a running diary of every experience so that in the end they could refer to it in judging the school along the lines of intellectualism, sociability, and athletic and school interest.

One of the chief details that aided Jay in his hoax on Stuart's fraternity, Theta Delta Chi, was a ping-pong tournament in which the house was then engaged. Using this as a medium for conversation, Jay was able to convince some suspicious "brothers" of his supposed identity.

One fellow in particular was so convinced that Jay was able to play him in Stuart's place for the fraternity elimination, and he never knew the difference. "Fortunately," Jay said, "I lost, for otherwise I would have faced other fraternity opponents who might have guessed the switch."

Both boys worked on their opposite newspapers for the week. The managing editor of the Williams, Record even said to Jay; "You know; Stu, you're getting to look so much; more like your brother." Jay, however, was able to brush this suspicion aside.

Stuart tells of similar experiences occurring at Wesleyan. A fellow in Jay's dorm suspected Stuart immediately, but the latter continued playing his part as Jay. After frequent conversations in which Stuart was able to prove he knew all necessary information (previously obtained from Jay) the boy apologized for ever believing the switch could take place.

Perhaps the funniest episode resulting from the switch was Jay's interview with Williams' Dean of Admissions, Frederic Copeland. When the Dean first saw Jay he yelled in jest: "Hi, Stu, how's that twin brother of yours? You know even if he wanted to transfer here, we wouldn't let him. We don't admit any dumb-bells from Wesleyan." Jay quickly retorted that he felt his brother was satisfied where he was. Finally after a long conversation in which Jay was able to obtain information on Williams' "excellent" incoming class, he let Copeland in on the secret.

Among the extra-curricular activities attended, Jay recalls primarily Stuart's glee club rehearsal when he was forced to sight-read without any detection. In addition he attended a committee luncheon in Stuart's place and discussed means of fostering better relations between the college and the infirmary.[4]

Jay and Stuart also wrote articles for *The Argus* about their experiences. Jay had some pointed commentary about Williams: "I noticed at once a slight variance in the amount of emphasis placed on certain aspects of college life. Williams does seem to lack an interest in the intellectual. The Williams student does not seem to want to learn merely for learning sake." He added that the Williams student "tends to think of his studies as a duty imposed by his school in order to pass and not as an introduction into interesting subjects and higher ideas on life." By contrast, Stuart noted that Wesleyan students tended to maximize their time in the library, which he found unsettling.

Student government

The campus switch with Stuart was just one of Jay's many extracurricular activities at Wesleyan. He was on the golf team and he wrote articles for *The Argus*, eventually serving as the paper's associate editor. He was also very active in his fraternity.

His interest in politics began when he campaigned for his uncle to get elected attorney general of Delaware. Thus it was no surprise that Jay would eventually seek office himself. He ran for student body vice president the spring of his junior year and as part of his campaign he proposed an "Educational-Directed Studies Program." He wanted to help provide intellectual enrichment to Wesleyan students by having them read literature, study foreign languages, and pursue science. His platform also called for giving students one week of no classes before final exams. Jay's opponent, Bruce Dow – a good friend and also a former resident of So-Est – put forward a campaign with ideas that *The Argus* characterized as addressing "basically short-range, student-centered problems."[5]

In comparing the Levy plan and the Dow plan, *The Argus* editors wrote that, "We tend to support the more ambitious, long-range approach offered in the Levy platform. We believe, simply, that this outlook better serves the needs of a fast-changing university community such as Wesleyan's."

Alas, both candidates felt that *The Argus* had mispresented their positions and they co-signed a letter to the paper's editor declaring that,

> If the Argus wishes to give an evaluation of the candidates' platforms it should describe them accurately; and 2) If the Argus then wishes to present its own point of view, it should concentrate on issues and not on personalities.[6]

(In a sign of just how enmeshed Jay was with campus affairs, when his letter to *The Argus* was published, he was also a member of *The Argus* editorial staff.)

It was a civil campaign – Jay gave talks at fraternities and the John Wesley Club and appeared on the campus radio station – with one exception. One of Jay's posters was defaced with a swastika. The incident was an awakening that even Wesleyan was not free of bigoted views. "It was my first exposure to antisemitism at Wesleyan," recalls Jay. "I was quite upset."

In the end, Jay prevailed, winning 262 votes, while Dow, his opponent, finished with 230.[7] And the student Senate later adopted Jay's campaign proposal related to greater intellectual enrichment.

Fraternity life

Wesleyan was all male during Jay's time there and fraternities loomed large on campus – 70-80 percent of freshmen would join ("pledge").[8] It was an era when *The Argus* would publish the names of the women being brought to fraternity parties, as well as their hosts.[9]

In the spring of his freshman year, Jay joined Alpha Chi Rho, which was often referred to as simply "Crow." Many of its members were singers, and in the fall of 1958 four of them – all enrolled at Wesleyan at the time – formed a group called The Highwaymen. They became "major recording stars" wrote *The Argus*.[10] They appeared on the Ed Sullivan show and a song of theirs, "Michael, Row the Boat Ashore," was #1 on the charts in the summer of 1960. Another member of the fraternity, Douglas Bennet, who was one year ahead of Jay, would go on to have a distinguished career in public service: he served in the State Department and as president of National Public Radio. From 1995-2007, he was president of Wesleyan.

Jay had several close friends in the fraternity and had many of his meals there. They were prepared by an Irish woman, known to everyone as "Mrs. McNally," who Jay recalls as "being like a mother to many in the house." Following each meal, the members would sing songs together, reflecting the reputation of Wesleyan as being "the singing college of New England." After the meal, they would often end up playing bridge, poker and other card games. The fraternity's older members provided advice, such as what courses to take and how to handle academic pressure.

Jay was an active member of Alpha Chi Rho and it occupied a prominent place in his college experience. During his junior and senior years, he helped organize cocktail parties for Wesleyan professors, who would then lead discussions focused on academia and everyday life. His experience in the fraternity also provided an early lesson in leadership and how to handle bigotry.

Alpha Chi Rho had been founded in 1895 at nearby Trinity College in Hartford, with an explicitly religious charter. Members would be drawn "from among Christians only," read its guiding principles. In 1954, the fraternity's Wesleyan chapter asked the national organization to remove that language, but it was only modified, to say that members would consider Jesus of Nazareth their moral exemplar. And according to *The Argus*, "the national organization retained a secret policy that not only restricted membership to Christians, but also excluded African Americans."[11]

In June 1957, a few Wesleyan members of Alpha Chi Rho met with officers of the fraternity's national organization to try to persuade them to modify the rules on eligibility. Those officers told the fraternity that its black and Jewish members needed to be purged. Failure to comply, said the officers, would lead to the members being evicted from the house.

The fraternity took no action and by the fall of 1957 its new members were being initiated without taking the official pledge.[12] A year later, the national organization announced it was suspending every Wesleyan member of Alpha Chi Rho.[13] This led to Jay and his fellow members dropping their affiliation with the national chapter and renaming the fraternity the "Black Walnut Club," which was the name of their eating club.

Amid this turmoil, Jay was elected president in the spring of 1959, his junior year. Soon thereafter, he and two of his brothers (Don Hinman and Gus Napier) met with national officials of Alpha Chi Rho in New York to discuss the suspension of Wesleyan members. An Alpha Chi Rho executive also met with Wesleyan alumni from the fraternity to discuss reinstating the chapter, which had been suspended after failing to include the discriminatory clauses from its initial ritual for new members.[14]

When these meetings didn't lead to any resolution, Jay attended the national convention of Alpha Chi Rho, in Columbus, Ohio. He was excited to make the trip – to get there, he took his first ride in an airplane – but he also knew the meeting could be contentious. It was an unlikely coincidence that the fraternity's organizers assigned him to a room with another Jew, Richard Levy, from Dartmouth. A group of young men later came to the room, having been told they could see boys with horns sprouting from their heads (a well-known trope for Jewish people).

At the meeting, Jay and Dick advocated for the fraternity being open to people of all races and religions. Their proposal was put to a vote, and in Jay's memory he and Dick were the only ones to support it. "I was convinced at that point that the Wesleyan chapter was going to need to separate itself from the national chapter," recalls Jay.

In September 1959, at the first Wesleyan chapter meeting in Middletown following this episode, Jay made the case for prohibiting discrimination among the fraternity's members. And he proposed that the house drop its association with the national chapter and adopt a new name. When it was put to a vote, it passed unanimously. The fraternity needed a new name, and Jay brainstormed with one of his fraternity brothers, Bob Patricelli. Having studied Latin for four years in high school, Jay suggested the fraternity call itself *Esse Quam Videri*, which is from Cicero and translates as, "To be, rather than to seem." "That name certainly summarized the experience with Alpha Chi Rho," recalls Jay. It was immediately adopted.

With this new identity, the fraternity thrived and was a hub of revelry, academic achievement, and social consciousness. In the 1960 presidential election, just 28 percent of EQV members reported voting for Nixon – the lowest percentage of any Wesleyan fraternity. (Beta and Delta Tau Delta recorded the highest level of support for Nixon – 70 percent.[15])

After graduating, some members of the fraternity established scholarship programs to provide support for young Wesleyan students who wanted to volunteer in less developed countries. But fraternities started to decline in popularity and when a fire ravaged EQV in December 1967 it was taken over by the university. Today, the building at 300 High Street, serves as the home of Wesleyan's Romance languages department.

Academics

Jay arrived at Wesleyan feeling his high school courses had prepared him well for a college curriculum. His freshman courses included biology, English, French, physics, and the humanities. In the English class, students had to write a short story each week, with a focus on different emotions. He recalls earning A's in all of his classes, with the exception of physics, which was reputed to be among the most challenging courses offered at Wesleyan.

In his sophomore year, Jay enrolled in six courses – the norm was four – but he continued to thrive, with fond memories of studying the history of art and the history of music. At the close of his sophomore year, he decided to major in biology and minor in French.

For four of his eight semesters at Wesleyan, Jay served as a teacher's assistant in science classes. The experience nurtured his interest in science, though he had another motive: he earned $75 per semester, which he applied toward his expenses at school – a way of showing gratitude toward his father, who was simultaneously paying for Stuart to attend Williams and later for their sister Ellen to attend Mount Holyoke.

During Jay's junior year, he read an article in a science journal written by a distinguished French scientist, Raymond Latarjet. The article suggested that cancer was due to a virus that remains silent within the cancer cell and then converts it into a malignant cell. It was a revolutionary idea and Jay was intrigued. The article led him to want to work in research to determine if this hypothesis could be correct. It also spoke to his excitement about scientific discovery. "That chance event, a *beshert* moment, became a major focus of the research I would later pursue," he recalled.

At the time, Jay was still undecided about whether to pursue a career in medicine or in diplomacy. He was auditing a class taught by an esteemed professor of government and social sciences, Sigmund Neumann. "I enjoyed looking up to people and having them mentor me," Jay recalled later. "I told Professor Neumann I was interested in medicine but also in being a diplomat and asked him what I should do." Neumann told him to focus on medicine but to keep politics and government as a hobby, and that, perhaps in the future, he would be able to blend his medical knowledge with his interest in international affairs. He advised Jay to keep international affairs as a hobby and one day "it could be part of your career." That prescient advice would later come true as Jay's AIDS research impacted health and public policy throughout the world.

Coming on the heels of Jay's interest in the work of Latarjet, the conversation helped convince Jay that he should apply to medical school. And he wanted to make the Latarjet idea the basis of his senior thesis, but no professor was available to serve as his advisor. Instead, he researched the role of oxygen in permitting the normal replication of cells and lack of oxygen favored the malignant cells.

Jay was determined to receive an "A" on his thesis. Doing so would enable him to be named a "Fellow" – a designation for graduating seniors who demonstrated strong academic performance across a range of disciplines.

One element of the project involved measuring the amount of oxygen being consumed by plants. Glass vessels were used to measure the oxygen content and they had to be handled with great care. One day, Jay was rushing through the measuring process – it was his 21st birthday and he wanted to get to a party his sister, Ellen, was giving at Mount Holyoke for him and Stuart. In the process, he broke one of the vessels. His advisor, who was known to have a bad temper, was so angry that he strongly criticized Jay and then later gave him a B+ on the project – which disqualified him from earning the "Fellow" designation. But his research was the basis of one of his first scientific papers.

But he didn't let this decision interfere with his non-science interests. During his senior year, he took a class on great writers and another on art. In the latter course, he was able to do oil paintings – he donated one of them, of his childhood tree hut, to Wesleyan. This interest in art was nurtured as well by Jay's friendship with a husband-and-wife team, Heinrich and Elizabeth Schwartz, both of whom were Holocaust survivors. They played a role in mentoring Jay in his senior year at Wesleyan and played an important part in having him appreciate the Rembrandt lithograph collection that was in Wesleyan's Davidson Art Center.

* * *

During Jay's time at Wesleyan, a professor of psychology, Karl Hagan, would give incoming freshmen a questionnaire to gauge their overall knowledge. Jay scored in the lowest 10 percent of his class. Hagan also gave the test to seniors as they were on the verge of graduating. This time, Jay scored in the top 10 percent of his class. And he graduated magna cum laude. "That was a tribute to the Wesleyan education I received," recalls Jay.

That improvement in knowledge is emblematic of the way in which Jay grew and thrived during his four years at Wesleyan, showing resilience after an unhappy first semester. And he benefited both inside and outside the classroom. He was one of three students nominated for the William Day Leonard award, which went to the student who best exemplified character and campus citizenship.[16] "There was nothing in my Wesleyan experience that I regretted, and there was so much that I valued," he recalls. "I had an incredible group of friends and faculty who gave me unlimited support."

"My experiences at Wesleyan," says Jay, 65 years after graduating, "reflect a life of intellectual exposure and scientific challenge – and an acceptance that ideas can eventually be valuable as mediators of a career. Wesleyan helped take the naïve thoughts and ambitions of a well-educated but somewhat unsophisticated student and transform those thoughts and ambitions into dreams that could be channeled toward important projects in international health."

Those dreams would have come to have far-reaching implications for people throughout the world. And the path to realizing them would be enabled by the next chapter in Jay's life: becoming a medical student at Columbia University.

Chapter 3

Apprendre – et Vivre

(Learning – and Living)

As Jay completed his senior year at Wesleyan, he was accepted at Columbia's medical school – and intended to enroll that fall. But one of his French professors, Alex Szogyi, encouraged him to apply for a Fulbright fellowship to spend a year in Paris. Intrigued by the idea, and wanting to improve his spoken French, Jay applied. He secured a Fulbright travel grant and a French government fellowship, for study in Paris, starting in September. Although he wasn't informed until late August, he was very excited about the opportunity. And news of the fellowship reached the *Wilmington Journal*, the city's afternoon newspaper, which published a short article about it the day before Jay was scheduled to depart.

While Stuart was going to be in Paris during the summer, traveling with friends, Jay opted to work that summer in Wilmington at two racehorse tracks as well as the state highway department (he secured the latter job through his uncle, H. Albert Young, who was Delaware's attorney general). The money earned from these jobs would serve him well for the year in Europe.

While in Paris, Stuart stopped in at the Fulbright office to inquire about the status of Jay's fellowship. He learned that Jay was going to be assigned to Tours, a university town famous for its French studies. Stuart thought Paris would be a better fit, so he requested that the program officials switch Jay to a Paris-based science laboratory. The request was approved (a *beshert* moment), which resulted in Jay working at the Faculty de Science in Orsay, a 20-minute train ride from Paris, where he studied the mechanism of regeneration in the flatworm Planaria. His preceptor was Tomas Lender, a well-respected biologist in France. Jay was surprised to be assigned this topic, as he had no background in it, but he knew Lender had been a student of Etienne Wolff, a well-respected and well-known French biologist.

In early September, Jay's parents took him to New York so he could board a ship – the Queen Mary – that would take him to France. The trip took about a week and there were several days of rough weather. The Fulbright students gathered on the ship's top deck to try to minimize their sea sickness. Jay can still recall climbing three sets of stairs in one step as the boat rocked up and down and from side to side.

When the Queen Mary finally reached Le Havre, the students disembarked and were taken by bus to the center of Paris. "My first memory is of the wide Avenue of the Champs Elysses and flowers blooming at both ends. I couldn't believe how beautiful it was," recalls Jay.

In Paris, Jay was given a dorm room at the Cite Universitaire but was quickly moved to be with students from Italy in the Maison de l'Italie. "I think looking Italian was the reason for this assignment," recalls Jay. This was another *beshert* moment. He was happy about this mistake since he wanted to avoid English and be immersed in French. Despite studying the language for seven years, he was struggling with conversations. And he did not want to be housed with Americans. Alas, when university officials discovered the mistake, they insisted he be reassigned to live with other Americans. Jay appealed to the Fulbright office in Paris and they agreed to let him live in a local apartment – and gave him an extra dollar a week to do so.

That was the turning point in his Paris experience. He found a room, for 5 francs (equivalent to about one dollar) per night, in the Hotel du

Grand Balcon, at the corner of Rue Dauphne and Rue Mazarine. It was in the center of the Latin Quarter and near Place de L'Odeon in the 6th district, an old section of Paris. It was a 5th floor walkup and had no shower and no toilet. "Even so," recalls Jay, "I was in ecstasy. I would walk outside and be enthralled that I was living in Paris on my own. Being in the hotel changed my life and my experience in Paris." The hotel's low price was also a blessing because Jay's father didn't approve of his year in Paris and refused to provide any financial support. His mother would occasionally send $5-$10 to supplement the monthly Fulbright stipend of $100.

But the experience in the hotel had one downside: Jay did not wash his hair for six months. When he finally did so, during a trip to London, the barber marveled at how filthy it had become and marched him around the salon so everyone could get a look.

Jay ate many of his meals at student restaurants in Paris for 2-3 francs, but he found them unappetizing. Once, a short time after his arrival in Paris, he found a white button in his food. When he approached the manager about this apparent lack of attention to the food, hundreds of the restaurant's patrons shouted, "*Viva Le Roi*" ("Long Live the King"). Jay was named "king" for that day and was asked to name a queen (he chose the first girl he saw). While the meaning of this spectacle was a mystery to Jay (it may have been on All Kings Day), it was a *beshert* moment, signaling that his luck had changed. "It was an amazing occurrence," he recalls. "It made me feel welcomed and changed my feelings for Paris. While I had been feeling some loneliness, this little episode dispelled that loneliness and made me feel accepted as a Parisian student. It seemed like it was meant to happen."

The money Jay earned from the three jobs in Wilmington gave him the financial cushion to purchase a car – for the equivalent of about $2,500

– just a month after arriving in France. He settled on a green Renault Fluoride convertible. "I loved the color," recalls Jay. He named the car "Esperance," which in French means "hope."

A few days after the button episode, Jay drove his car to the French Riviera, taking with him Margot Callahan, a tall American girl studying French in Paris and David, another American student. Joining them on the ride was his Italian student friend, Guccio Visentini. They left Guccio at a bus station at the border of France and Italy to find his way home. "I felt a bit guilty about this," recalled Jay. "But I later learned European students were very adept at finding solutions and he made it home without incident." Jay continued on to Spain and Portugal – a two-week trip that resulted in friendships that endured for decades. One of the highlights was staying at a farm, for no fee, and sleeping in a haystack.

Soon after returning to Paris, Jay met a young blond-haired English girl named Judy Wheaton at the symphony. The next day, after learning that she was babysitting for a French family, he surprised her by showing up at the house. She was pleased to see him and they spoke for about two hours. She then returned to England but said she would visit him in Israel the following summer. "I was smitten by Judy and hoped to see her again," recalls Jay. But she ultimately chose to travel in Israel with a different group of students. "It was one of the first disappointments in my social life."

Jay had another friend in Paris, an 18-year-old French girl named Annie Landes. A Wesleyan professor had recommended he contact her family upon arriving in Paris, and after doing so, he drove to the suburbs where Annie lived with her parents. Jay and Annie quickly developed a strong friendship. They traveled together (in Paris and beyond), attended movies together, and explored restaurants. One night, they slept on the banks of the Seine. It was in the same spot where the lead actress from the

Jules et Jim film, Jeanne Moreau, fell into the river. "That was a somewhat romantic episode I wished to experience," recalls Jay. They also went to a concert featuring Edith Piaf, the famous French cabaret singer, and explored local shops and tourist spots. But their contact ceased six months later when a boyfriend, whom Annie later married, asked her to stop seeing Jay.

Amid Jay's travels and socializing, he continued to work with Lender and became acquainted with the fields of embryogenesis and regeneration. Some of the work was tedious, so he pursued a more ambitious experiment: he anesthetized more than 100 planaria (collected a short distance from the lab) by submerging them in ice water. After placing them on a wax slab that he created, he took a sharp knife and cut groups of planaria near the head or the tail and then placed the pieces in bowls containing water and various concentrations of metals. His objective was to determine the effect of metals on regeneration. While he recalls that his observations were "not that interesting," he told Lender he had done over 100 experiments in one week. Lender then shared this news with his laboratory workers, to try to motivate them to be more productive saying that, "our American visitor conducted 100 experiments this week." That did not endear Jay to his coworkers.

One of the first research projects Lender assigned to him was to take a week and find planaria in the countryside. On his first day, Jay found all the planaria he needed under rocks in a stream near the lab. This left him with a full week to do whatever he wanted. And while research labs typically worked Monday to Saturday, Lender did not ask him to work on Saturdays, thinking that Jay observed the Sabbath. Jay didn't correct him, which gave him an extra day for exploration and leisure every week.

Jay's life in France was soon full of adventures. He often took his car for drives in the countryside. He enjoyed the stops he made on the short trips and the various bridges crossing the Seine where he began to do charcoal sketches. It made him think of the famous French artists who emphasized the Seine during the Impressionist era.

One weekend, he drove to Alsace Lorraine and woke up very early on a Monday because he had a meeting with Lender that morning. But he fell asleep at the wheel and the car jumped a ditch and rolled over. The Renault had no seat belts but – incredibly – Jay was not ejected from the car. In fact, he had no injuries, even though one of his shoes was found 100 feet away. People who saw the accident rushed to help him, and they gave him wine to calm his nerves. When the police arrived they accused him of drunk driving. The father of his friend Annie came to the rescue after Jay contacted him and said the accident occurred after Jay had tried to adjust his contact lens, which was partly true. He also arranged for Jay's car to be towed and persuaded the authorities the accident wasn't Jay's fault. Jay soon received a brand-new Renaut from his insurance company and continued to use it in travels in Paris or to the countryside. "I felt someone was protecting me," says Jay. "And Annie's dad intervening on my behalf was certainly a *beshert* moment."

During Jay's time in Paris, he frequented bars like Old Navy or the Left Bank in the Latin quarter. While there, he loved to drink Ricard, a licorice-flavored aperitif. That also seemed to calm his nerves. He would chat with writers and poets, some of them well-known, such as Arthur Adamov and the Lebanese playwright Georges Schehadé, who wrote in French. Jay worked on translating the plays of Schehadé into English, but was disappointed he could not get the translations published. Nonetheless, the experience "made me feel that I was really living the life of a Parisian writer."

Jay's parents came to Paris in April 1961 and barely recognized him: he had replaced his glasses with contact lenses, he had long hair, and he wore a scarf around his neck. "I looked like a regular French guy," recalls Jay. "I even started thinking in French." This became apparent when one day while in conversation with a friend and the friend's cousin. Upon telling the cousin that he was disappointed not to be thinking in French, she told him he was wrong, given the speed with which he was speaking. Jay became convinced that she was right and soon thereafter he became very comfortable thinking and speaking in French.

When Jay's fellowship was ending, he wanted to stay in France for another year, as he was thoroughly enjoying his experience. "I mostly used my time to meet people, improve my French, and immerse myself in French culture and life" he recalls. The Fulbright fellowship staff approved an extension, but Jay's Dad objected. "He told me if I spent another year in France, it will be just like the year I'd already had," recalls Jay. "He said I should return when I was older, as I would have a different experience." After a few weeks of reflection, Jay said goodbye to his friends and prepared to start medical school at Columbia. That proved to be the right decision.

Jay says that his experiences in Paris "played a role in my maturity" and helped him see the value in meeting a wide variety of people. He remained in contact with several friends he made while in Paris – and some of them he still sees today. Above all, recalls Jay, "my days in Paris contributed to my appreciation for the arts – drawing, painting, writing, living as a relatively poor student mindful of expenses."

Chapter 1

A Medical School Education –
Inside and Outside the Classroom

When Jay arrived at Columbia in September 1961, he stood out from other students. He was a year older than most of his classmates and he wasn't obsessed with his grades. "I really wanted to understand everything that was being taught," he recalls. Some professors would have their lectures recorded by the students, with a transcript available following the lecture. The transcript would then be shared with a note-taking group. Jay refused to participate in this. "I thought it was kind of cheating to have the notes taken by scribes from the class. As a result, I wasn't in the top of my class academically," he recalls, "but it didn't bother me. I was a solid B student and I was learning the material. I particularly enjoyed the introduction to immunology and virology." In retrospect, says Jay, "I think I was rather naïve and should have taken advantage of anything that would help me master my medical school classes."

Jay had an intellectual awakening in his second year at Columbia. He sought out a lab that was studying the hidden viruses in bacterial cells – a topic covered in the Latarjet article that he had discovered while browsing through cancer research journals in the Wesleyan library. He volunteered to join the laboratory of Herbert Rosenkranz to study lysogeny in bacteria, a process by which bacterial viruses silently infect bacteria and affect their function. Jay worked in the lab during the evenings and interacted with Rosenkrantz and others in the lab, when possible during the day, which strengthened his interest in research.

He liked being involved in novel studies in microbiology while simultaneously taking the required courses for medical school. He continued to work in the lab through his third and fourth years of medical school. That research led him to discover that a recently developed chemical drug, hydroxyurea (HU), was unique in blocking DNA synthesis but not RNA synthesis. Rosencrantz had obtained the drug to see if it would activate bacterial viruses from a latent state. By surprise, Jay showed that lysogenic bacteria grown in the presence of HU became larger without any major effect on their replicative state – nor lysogeny. This activity also explained why he found an increase in protein production in his cultures treated with HU without a change in number of individual bacteria recovered after treatment. The latter was proven by plating the treated cells on blood agar plates. The results showed the same number of bacteria colonies in the HU cultures as appeared at the beginning of the experiment.

This observation with the new drug was unexpected and gave Jay the opportunity to see how making a novel observation can be exhilarating – and also how it could lead to more research opportunities. The discovery led to some important articles on this unique finding, which was a strong way to start his research with HU and lysogenic bacteria. The drug answered a later challenge facing the laboratory of an NIH scientist, Robert Huebner (which Jay joined after medical school): how to make lots of protein using a major function of a bacterium. "I was viewed as something of a heroic researcher after that," recalls Jay.

During the summer between his first and second year of medical school, Jay went to Israel and lived part-time on a kibbutz. He volunteered to work with a social medicine doctor, Sidney Kark, in a small village established for recent immigrants from North Africa. They lived in huts, which were made using asbestos, because it wouldn't burn. The village was called "Asbestosonim." The toxic effect of asbestos (it can induce mesotheliomas) was not known then. The inhabitants eventually had to be moved to other places.

As a clinical assistant in the village, Jay would help patients who were afflicted with a wide range of conditions. He learned various phases of medical care including clinical services, rehabilitation, physical therapy, social therapy, and occupational therapy. "The experience taught me about the difficulty in working with patients who spoke a different language and who often had poor health and little access to medical care," recalls Jay. "It also convinced me that I was also interested in clinical issues, particularly in international health. It was another awakening and a *beshert* experience." He was particularly pleased to work with the patient who had had a stroke and had injuries to his leg. "It was a great thrill, at the end of the summer, to walk with this man in a parade that ended at his synagogue."

During that summer, he also provided primary care for immigrants who had moved from the Atlas Mountains in Morocco. The immigrants identified as Jewish and had lived in caves in Morocco. They were given housing in a village outside Jerusalem, but over time they dug tunnels to replicate the caves from their past and began living there. But at the same time, their young children were bicycling outside. "I had to congratulate the Israelis, who just wanted the immigrants to be immersed in modern life," recalls Jay.

After returning to Columbia for his second year of medical school, Jay was admitted into Columbia's School of International and Public Affairs (SIPA). He was recommended for this program by John Macy, the vice president of Wesleyan who had become a good friend and advisor. Being part of SIPA addressed Jay's need to feel involved with international issues, and doing so through the prism of medicine. "I was the only medical school student at SIPA and I cherished the opportunities to interact with people from Columbia's many different schools, including literature, law, journalism, and music," recalls Jay. His thesis focused on major features of international health, emphasizing disease prevention and care. "SIPA helped me get through medical school," recalls Jay. "I benefited from my interaction with students from different disciplines. It kept me intellectually stimulated and encouraged my training in academic medicine."

Between his second and third year of medical school, Jay researched lysogeny with Giuseppe and Elizabeth Bertani while working for two months at the Karolinska Institute in Stockholm. Seeking to maximize the experience, he set out to learn Swedish and found a professor of anesthesiology at Columbia, Jan Gyessing, to serve as his instructor, with weekly sessions. In the lab that summer, he insisted that he only be spoken to in Swedish. He would try his Swedish when talking to local women at social clubs, but these encounters often began when Jay was seated. Upon standing up to dance, he found that he was shorter than many of the women. On a brighter note, Jay befriended several Swedes, and he has remained friends with two of them from Stockholm – Per Hendrickson and Leif Moeller – to this day.

Jay has always believed in the idea, first promulgated by a psychiatrist in England, that energy expended in one direction will come back in another and he channeled that theory to direct his approaches to find a summer position. He wrote to scientists throughout the world but initially only received rejections. But he was pleasantly surprised when he received a letter from Louisiana State University (LSU) asking if he was interested in a fellowship.

The fellowship was supposed to be in South America, but Jay wanted to go to Africa – and he convinced LSU to allow him to do so. His focus was the potential role of viruses in cancer – citing the article by Raymond Latarjet that he had discovered while at Wesleyan. The fellowship let him work with Denis Burkitt, who had described lymphomas in young children in Africa who lived in areas under 5,000 feet in elevation, receiving 20 inches of rainfall and with mild temperatures spanning from 25 to 60° F, all of which was suggestive of insect-borne agents.

Jay spent much of his time working at the East African Virus Research Institute in Entebbe, Uganda, and that experience deepened his understanding of diagnostic virology. His research continued the study at the Institute conducted by Alexander Haddow and Tom Bell, which revealed antibodies to reoviruses in sera from Burkitt patients. (That discovery sparked research on these RNA viruses when he returned to Columbia.)

Jay was fortunate to be associated with the Mulago Hospital in Kampala. He rotated in other medical groups and greatly benefited from the clinical experience. Jay also treated patients at outdoor clinics, where locals lined up at a makeshift "clinic under a tree" and shared their symptoms, many of which were respiratory and tied to measles. During his first week participating in the clinic, he was chastised by a nurse for using a stethoscope. She reminded him that there were over 500 patients to see that morning and that he shouldn't be using an instrument to look for features of a disease. "You need to use your eyes and brain and come up with the most logical medical cause," she told him. They quickly learned that most of his patients had respiratory problems from secondary measles. There were also cases of smallpox and tetanus, which Jay knew he would not see in the United States.

Jay was fortunate in being associated with Mulago Hospital in Kampala, a first-rate institution at the time and where he met Denis Burkitt. He told him how much his work on lymphoma influenced his desire to study virology and to find a solution for cancer. He joined Burkitt in a couple of his operations but did not otherwise have much contact with him. On visits to Kampala in recent years, Jay saw that the hospital's facilities had severely declined. Lacking support from medical programs in England, the elevators did not work and patients in beds had to be carried down the steps to go to rooms for radiation or follow-up studies.

One of his memorable experiences unfolded when Jay was returning from a Catholic hospital clinic visit in the north of Kampala. He encountered a circumcision ceremony of a boy about 13 years old. There was a crowd and the procedure – part of a "coming of age" ritual – was done without anesthesia. The young boy simply had to tolerate the pain, without wincing, and to try to blunt it he drank a lot of local wine. Jay was assigned by tribal members to the front row to watch. Afterwards, the boy was rushed to the hospital, as the knife used for circumcision was not sterilized and had apparently been stored in a leather satchel for months.

At the Institute in Entebbe, Jay helped to euthanize monkeys in order to get access to their kidneys. He cultured their renal cells, which were sensitive to many viruses. One evening, Haddow came to see him at one of the outdoor clinics. He asked Jay if he could help with the collection of mosquitoes that might carry the virus causing Burkitt's lymphoma. Jay immediately accepted. They were trying to see what viruses were carried by the mosquitoes and to explore the connection with reoviruses and other potential infectious agents.

Jay was paired with a young African student. They were told to climb a tree in the forest at dusk and expose their legs, as doing so would attract the mosquitoes that carry viruses. But only live mosquitoes could be studied, so Jay and the student had to resist the temptation to swat the mosquitoes that landed on them. "The student was much better at this than I was," recalls

Jay. I had many fewer mosquitoes.

Jay's research in Uganda also involved looking for malaria parasites in placentas from African women. Work on that project was directed by Derrick and Patrice Jelliffe, who were pediatricians stationed in Uganda and part of the scientific committee of the LSU program. Jay used this opportunity to study Burkitt's lymphoma. He would go to villages and get permission from the local tribal leader to take blood samples from a variety of young children, some of whom had Burkitt's lymphoma. This study enabled him to collect the valuable source of sera that would later be useful in linking the Epstein Barr virus to Burkitt's lymphoma.

Near the end of his time in Uganda, the grandmother of a young boy whom Jay had bled told the chieftain that Jay was drinking the blood from the children. "The chief, who had given me permission for the bleed, immediately changed his tune and pretended he did not know anything about the study," recalls Jay. Some teachers said that the war drums were being beaten and the Secretary of Health had to appear on Uganda television to explain the situation. Fortunately, Sidney Kark, whom Jay knew from Israel, was also in Uganda and took Jay to his home. The US embassy advised him to leave the country immediately, which he did, with assistance from the Israeli embassy.

Jay flew to Kenya to meet Stuart, who was also in Africa studying tropical disease. Jay was assigned to study tropical skin ulcers in the town of Loitokitok, which was at the foot of Mount Kilimanjaro. Jay noticed this skin problem after seeing the children walk to school and pass through fields packed with shrubs containing sharp needles. The needles led to bleeding, which attracted swarms of flies. Jay obtained a portable incubator in which the heat was generated by a candle. He used blood agar plates and took cultures from the ulcers in small children and then encouraged the students to wash the cuts on their legs every morning when they came to the school. (Jay also encouraged the schoolmasters to introduce soap and water in classrooms.) That sharply reduced the number of flies swarming around the young students and the onset of new skin lesions.

During his day in the small Kenyan village, Jay was given the cabin of the public health officer for the region. While there, he met a guide who arranged for him to climb Mount Kilimanjaro and who was the same guide Ernest Hemingway used when visiting Kenya. They started the hike early in the morning and the barefoot guide carried equipment and food on his back. Jay had no trouble on the hike until the final 1,000 yards. He desperately needed oxygen and would take two steps forward and one step back. "I could not shout or speak to my guide so I used sign language to try to say I could not make it," recalls Jay.

But they soldiered on, spending one night in a tent, and arrived at the top of Kilimanjaro by 1 p.m. A book was there, signed by successful climbers. Jay gathered his strength and wrote in it, "Never Again." The guide gave him a wreath of dried flowers taken from the top of the mountain to show to others that he had completed the climb.

For the descent, Jay ran down the trail, which took about 3-4 hours. He then went to the home of his Indian guide, where he had a spicy Indian meal. He developed gastritis, which he believed was triggered by the combination of a low oxygen level and spicy food. He asked for milk, which needed to be boiled because it was from cows that could have been infected with TB. The strong stomach pain endured for another 2-3 days.

This four-month experience was his introduction to tropical medicine and deepened his interest in international health issues. "It was *beshert*," recalls Jay. "One of the reasons I was enthusiastic about studying AIDS, which was an international disease, was my experiences in Uganda and

Kenya"

Jay enjoyed his time in Africa so much that he flew back to New York just in time to accept his rotation in surgery at St. Luke's Hospital. Deeply fatigued, he noticed a thin elevation of the skin near his right ankle. The elevation looked like it was covering underground canals. A dermatologist inspected it and immediately opened the covering. Inside was a sleeve of eggs that would have been laid there by an insect. The dermatologist immediately removed them. "It was upsetting to have the insect eggs in my skin, but at the same time fascinating to see the long egg chain extracted from the canals," recalls Jay. "I had unwittingly brought Africa to New York."

During Jay's fourth year at Columbia, he worked in the diagnostic virology laboratory with his technician, Eru Tanabe. She was assigned to him as a teacher and coworker by Edward Curnen, a professor in the pediatrics department and director of the diagnostic virology unit. (Jay says Curnen and Tanabe played "important roles" in introducing him to diagnostic virology.) Jay was then given free range to do a variety of virology procedures conducted by Tanabe in the medical school's pediatric virus diagnostic laboratory. "That was my big *beshert* moment – the introduction to diagnostic virology," recalls Jay. "I learned various facets of growing and identifying different viruses by procedures, including hemagglutination, heme absorption, complement formation, and serologic neutralizations." Tanabe introduced him to the variety of cytopathic or biological changes in cells that were related to a particular virus, mostly linked to pediatric disease. (This research depended on measuring the effect of viruses and cultures at odd hours, which forced Jay to sleep in the lab on some occasions.)

Monkey kidney cells were highly sensitive for culturing suspected viruses. The latter assay was an embarrassing moment when Jay, after his return to Columbia, asked Curnen where the monkeys could be housed to obtain the kidneys for renal cells. They all had a big laugh when Jay learned that the cells were purchased already cultured from one of the commercial biologic laboratories.

With Tanabe's help, Jay continued his project with Burkitt's lymphoma. "My objective was to determine if I could confirm the increased presence of reovirus antibodies in sera from Burkitt's lymphoma patients in comparison to sera from healthy normal, African children," recalls Jay. They tested the antibodies to reovirus 1, 2, and 3 and found the increase in incidence primarily to antibodies to reovirus 3. To conduct these studies, Jay had a cot in the lab and had to take hourly readings for some of these assays. This was his introduction to the intricacies of viral diagnosis. (He later learned that his boss at NIH, Robert Huebner, slept in the lab during his experiences with viruses and often met people in pajamas at the start of the day.) The lab quickly recognized that the higher level of antibody could reflect the hospitalization of the Burkitt lymphoma patients they were studying. More specifically, the patients could have been infected in the hospital wards by reoviruses carried there by other children bitten by mosquitos. This suspicion soon became the truth.

Ironically, a husband-and-wife team of scientists at the University of Pennsylvania, Werner and Gertrude Henle, later determined that antibodies to the Epstein-Barr virus was strongly associated with Burkitt's lymphoma. They were later credited with finding the first human cancer virus.

They also determined that EBV was highly associated with infectious mononucleosis. That discovery was made by chance when one of their technicians came down with infectious mono and she had been used as a negative control for their studies of EBV. She was now positive for infection by the virus. This chance event also related in part to Jay's working as an intern at night in their lab looking for antibodies to EBV in Burkitt's lymphoma patients. The handlers had seen evidence of these antibodies using established lymphoid cell lines and they needed early lymphoma sera to establish their assay. In a visit to Columbia University to see their friend Hattie Alexander, who was a leading pediatric physician at the medical center, they noted their need for BL sera. Curnen and Alexander said that they were working directly with someone who just left Africa and had a collection of BL sera. That was Jay's introduction to the Henles, two of his heroes in virology. They were surprised to learn that his sister, Ellen, was doing research in their laboratory with one of their assistants, Kurt Paucher "Another *beshert* experience," notes Jay.

Jay's other experiences at medical school were not as stimulating as living in Africa and other parts of the world. "I didn't find medical school that demanding," he recalls, noting that he did make time for extracurricular activities with his fellow students. This included writing the songs for a theatrical production at the medical school and taking advantage of shows and museums in New York.

During his first year, Jay took other medical school students to see "Who's Afraid of Virginia Wolff?" by Edward Albee. In advance of attending the play, Jay wrote to Albee and told him of his interest in theater of the absurd and his friendship with the playwright Samuel Beckett (see Appendix 1). Albee responded and later treated the medical students to a session on acting and discussion on the theater of the absurd. "That visit," recalls Jay, "was one of the most memorable experiences I had while in medical school.

After graduating from Columbia, Jay started his internship and residency at the University of Pennsylvania. Stuart had recently completed his medical studies there, and Jay inherited some of his patients. Meanwhile, Stuart had started a residency and internship in New York. In that position, he was at Mount Sinai Hospital, where he interacted with students from Columbia whom Jay knew. In particular, he worked with Charlotte Friend, who had made a landmark discovery involving a mouse retrovirus that induced blood cancers in mice.

While at Penn, where his fellow interns soon called him "the Wistar fellow" (he was also affiliated with the Wistar Institute, a biomedical research center across the street from his clinic), Jay discovered that his earlier research on the role of reoviruses in lymphoma was incorrect. Instead, as described above, a herpes virus, known now as Epstein-Barr, was associated with this cancer. Jay worked on that project with Werner and Gertrude Henle. They were researching Burkitt lymphoma and asked Jay for blood samples he'd taken from people with the cancer. From there, a working relationship developed and they taught Jay how to use an immunofluorescence assay when doing virus antibody studies of Burkitt lymphoma patients. Their work resulted in a paper published in the *Journal of Microbiology*.

While researching this virus, Jay interacted with researchers and clinicians who had been involved with the training of Stuart as well as their sister, Ellen, who was also studying at University of Pennsylvania's Children's Hospital to become a researcher. Jay also enjoyed doing basic science studies with some of his medical students, such as showing that the serum of a woman with thyroid disease produced bulging of eyes in goldfish. Another high point came when he correctly diagnosed a woman with Sjogren's disease whose symptoms had been described in more than 15 charts and had a diagnosis that mystified doctors in multiple clinics.

Jay's research – particularly on Burkitt's lymphoma during this research positioned him to thrive in the next stage of his medical journey.

My work with Burkitt's lymphoma emphasized the fact that a virus could be closely associated with cancer and that it might not be a direct cause of cell transformation but could promote the cancer process. In terms of HIV research, this experience enabled me to appreciate the role of the immune system in enhancing the cancer process and in giving rise to the immune abnormalities in HIV infection. In both situations, a hyper-response of the immune system could also be the cause of the disease process.

Chapter 5

Work and Play in Washington, DC

Jay arrived in Washington, DC in September 1966 to work at the National Institutes of Health, the US government's medical research agency. He was hired into the highly competitive Associate Training Program (ATP), which was part of the Commissioned Corps of the United States Public Health Service. Jay and all others in this group carried out clinical duties and conducted bench research in the lab of a senior NIH scientist.

The ATP "had the pick of the best and brightest medical school graduates," according to an NIH history paper written several decades later. The paper noted that "the ATP proved to be an incredibly successful program, ultimately producing many of the top-notch physician-scientists of that generation."[17] Indeed, 10 individuals who served as clinical associates (CAs) went on to win Nobel Prizes: Harvey Alter, Richard Axel, Michael Bishop, Michael Brown, Alfred Gilman, Joseph Goldstein, Robert Lefkowitz, Ferid Murad, Stanley Prusiner, and Harold Varmus. Several decades later, one other clinical associate would achieve fame and notoriety for his leadership on trying to contain the Covid-19 virus: Anthony Fauci.

The clinical associates became known as the "Yellow Berets" – a sharp contrast to the Green Berets, who fought in Vietnam. "The Yellow Beret label implied cowardice," according to the NIH paper, "possibly because supporters of the war effort viewed the CAs as trying to stay out of harm's way." According to Jay, some of the CAs were, in fact, trying to avoid military service. But with so much success among the scientists in the group, "the designation of Yellow Beret eventually became a badge of honor."

Jay applied and was accepted to work in the lab of Robert Huebner, who was one of the world's leading virologists and chief of the Laboratory of Viral Diseases (LVD) of the National Institute of Allergy and Infectious Diseases (NIAID) at NIH. Working with Huebner, who welcomed Jay with a handwritten note, "assured that my experience would be worthwhile," recalls Jay. (Stuart was also at NIH as a "Yellow Beret," at the same time as Jay, working in a biochemical lab headed by Loretta Leive.)

It was a miracle that Jay even reached the NIH. While he was at Penn, the Public Health Service declared it wasn't going to accept him, given that he had suffered from osteomyelitis as a child. As noted earlier, that resulted in his left foot being smaller than his right foot (osteomyelitis curbed its growth). He was also left with a shrunken fourth toe (the one next to his little toe). That could have led to him being forced to serve in the armed services, which he didn't want to do. And the next day, he received a letter from the Army instructing him to report for initiation in eight months. "The prospect of going into battle in Vietnam was the greatest emotional trauma I've ever had," recalls Jay.

Searching for advice, he went to see the head of medicine at Penn, James Weingarden. He said he would fight for Jay, who had already been accepted by Huebner but had not yet started work at the NIH. Weingarden asked the new vice president at Penn, Luther Terry, who had previously served as US Surgeon General, to write a letter to the Army stating that Jay should be accepted in the Public Health Service. Several other department heads wrote on Jay's behalf and the pressure worked: Jay was granted admission to the Public Health Service. That was *beshert*.

Soon after starting at NIH, Huebner told Jay to stop researching the Epstein-Barr virus and switch to adenoviruses because he thought they might be involved with human cancers. Jay was able to draw on his hydroxyurea work from Columbia, telling Huebner, "If hydroxyurea makes a bacterium produce more protein but not divide, maybe hydroxyurea will cause the virus to make more and more protein but not destroy the cell, because the virus can't replicate." He was right.

For his NIH studies, Huebner farmed out Jay to a company, which is where this research was conducted. But given Jay's age, he didn't get credit for the discovery, which was the basis of a paper published in *Nature*. In an oral history, Jay recounted what happened next:

> The people at the company who had been working on this challenge for a long time became jealous. They started to bad-mouth me. I'm not really sure what they said, but I know that they said enough that Huebner took me off the project completely. I fortunately was still able to publish the paper that showed the effect of hydroxyurea. One man [a technician] even poisoned my animals. So all the things you hear about what can go on in labs can unfortunately be correct at times. So I'd say that was the second trauma in my life. The first was almost going to Vietnam and not NIH.[18]

When the technician poisoned animals Jay was using in research, Jay reported him. Huebner sided with the technician and then criticized Jay, telling him he was "worthless" and lucky to work in the lab. Jay refers to this as Huebner's "annihilation speech" (as he later learned from NIH colleagues). He was left rattled – and in tears. Huebner then invited Jay to dinner that night, Jay recalls, "but I was too upset to accept."

The episode could have prompted some researchers to resign. But Jay stayed and later learned that others who had worked in the lab had similar experiences with Huebner, which provided some modest comfort. Huebner eventually invited Jay to visit his family's farm in Maryland one Sunday afternoon – an invite that Jay treasured and an occasion he enjoyed.

Jay was soon transferred back to NIH, where he worked under Wally Rowe and Janet Hartley. This new assignment came about through the help of Mike Oxman, another yellow beret who had heard how Jay was treated at the company and convinced Wally Rowe to accept him in his group in building 5 of NIAID on the NIH campus.

Working with the Huebner group, Jay made another major discovery. Rowe, who was his boss, showed him a black mouse in a cage, which he said had a predilection to develop autoimmune disease and cancer. They knew that this NZB mouse had a virus that resembled the known animal RNA tumor viruses causing leukemia and sarcoma in mice. (These viruses have been termed RNA tumor viruses.) The NZB virus, detected by electron microscopy, could not be grown in the laboratory, according to the laboratory reports. Rowe told him, "Jay, this is your project. You have to get the virus out, and you're to figure out what it does."

Jay set out to show that the virus had biologic functions. To do so, he developed a technique that could demonstrate this NZB virus was infectious – he evaluated its ability to transfer a biologically transforming gene from one cell into a different cell. He demonstrated that the EM NZB tumor virus was able to transfer a transforming gene into a new cell. He succeeded in showing this tumor-inducing activity – but only when using rat cells as the recipient cells, not mouse cells. This unexpected discovery proved biologic activity of the NZB virus and also showed that the transfer could not be made into any mouse cells, including those from which the NZB virus originated.

"Demonstrating that a virus that comes from an NZB mouse won't go back into the same animal species was a very big discovery," recalls Jay. "It created a new paradigm in virology and put me on the map as a researcher." Indeed, Jay described his findings in a paper that was published in *Science*.[19]

This discovery also led to Jay introducing new terminology for mouse cells and tumor viruses. The viruses that grew only in mouse species and thus were different from NZB viruses were called "xenotropic" (*xenos*, a Greek word meaning "foreign" and *tropic*, a Greek word meaning "attractive to"), while those that grew in mouse cells were called "ecotropic" (*ecos*, a Greek word meaning "home"). Later, Murray Gardner from UC Davis found a wild mouse retrovirus that could infect mouse cells as well as foreign cells. They were named "amphotropic mouse retroviruses" (*amphos*, a Greek word meaning "both").

Jay benefited from his positive relationship with Huebner, whose stature stemmed from both his creative ideas and his control over a large amount of research money. When Jay left NIH in 1970, Huebner granted him $100,000 per year for a few years to search for xenotropic human viruses in placentas, since this tissue in mice had many diverse types of viruses. "Huebner was larger than life," recalls Jay. "He had a big personality and told great stories. He also never spoke ill of anyone. He was a great role model."

Jay also had a special relationship with Huebner's wife, Harriet. She was a strong ally and had a kinship with Jay, almost treating him as an adopted son. "I always knew Harriet had my back," recalls Jay "and I often considered her as family."

Reflecting on his time at NIH, Jay recalls a lot of hard work – he developed carpal tunnel syndrome from pipetting so much – but getting major papers published made it all worthwhile.

> I attribute my emergence as a virologist to my two years with Huebner. I learned how to interact with technicians, and lab and cell culture procedures, by following Hartley's style. I learned critical approaches to science and how to question scientific facts from Rowe, and I learned about the role of a senior scientist at NIH from Huebner. These three virologists gave me the background and intellectual curiosity I needed to become an independent scientist.

Socializing in the nation's capital

Jay had a demanding schedule at NIH, but he still found time to maintain an active social life. His annual salary was $10,000 – equivalent to nearly $100,000 today. Washington was much more affordable in the 1960s, and he and Stuart were able to rent a three-bedroom carriage house on P Street, NW in Georgetown – an upscale Washington neighborhood.

The two well-credentialed bachelors regularly attended black-tie events at embassies and hosted dinner parties in their home. Jay dated a woman who worked at the Embassy of Finland and she would give him as much vodka as he wanted for their parties. He and Stuart became "go-to" young men to show up at black-tie embassy parties.

They hosted an annual Columbus Day party at their carriage house. Each party featured a band and outdoor dancing in their courtyard. At one of them, they staged a reenactment of the fabled Jewish-themed musical, "Fiddler on the Roof," complete with a real fiddler on the roof of their home. Attendees were asked to sign a book when entering the party, and for kicks Jay and Stuart included the names of the President (Richard Nixon) and the Vice President (Spiro Agnew) as expected invitees.

"My time in Washington featured many of the most entertaining, influential, and rewarding experiences of my life," recalls Jay. "Those three years were among the best years of my life." When Jay celebrated his 85th birthday in New York, several of his friends from Washington were in attendance.

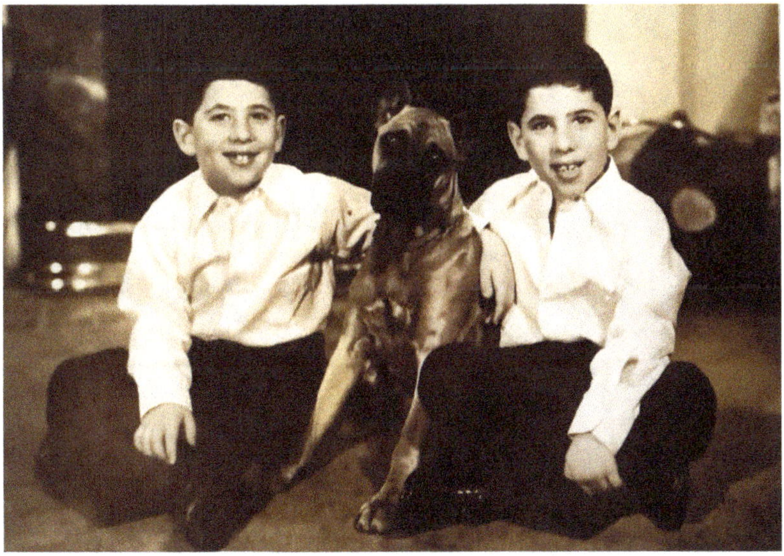

Stuart and Jay (right) with their pet dog, Connie, in the living room of their childhood home in Carrcroft, Delaware, 1944

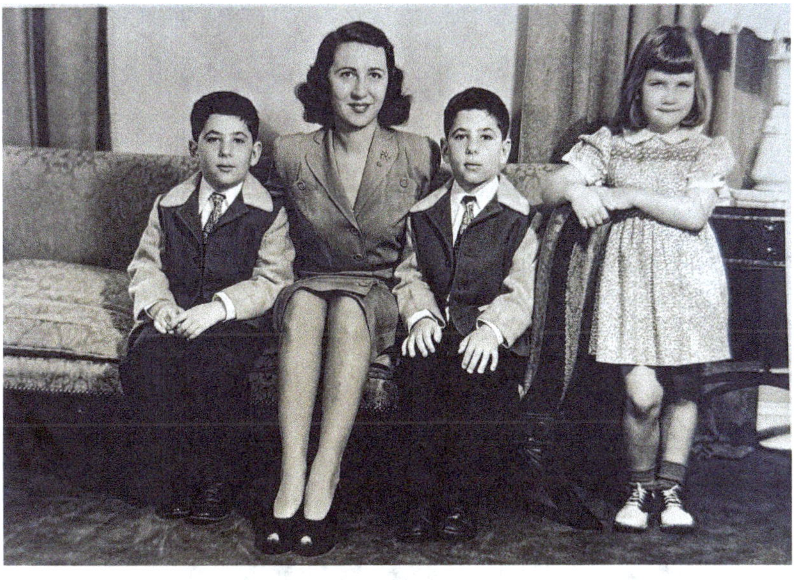

Stuart (left), Jay, and Ellen with their mother, Ruth, February 1, 1946

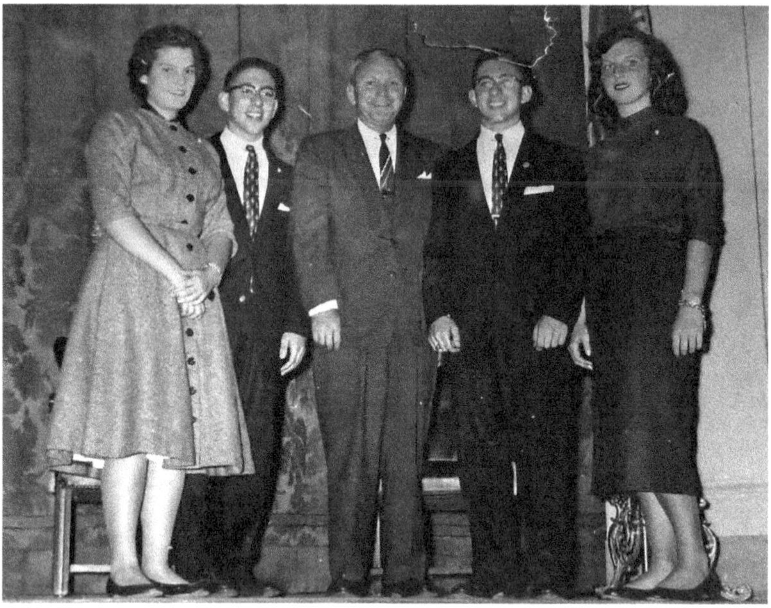

Delaware Governor Caleb Boggs with Stuart (right), Jay, and other high school Student Council officers, 1955

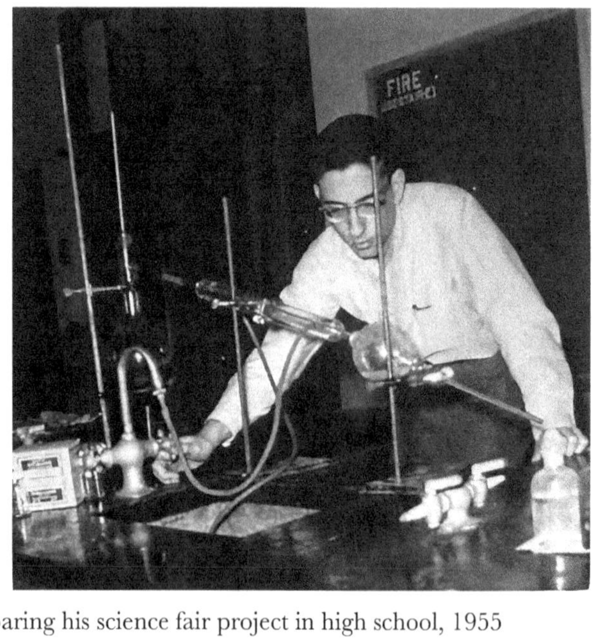

Jay preparing his science fair project in high school, 1955

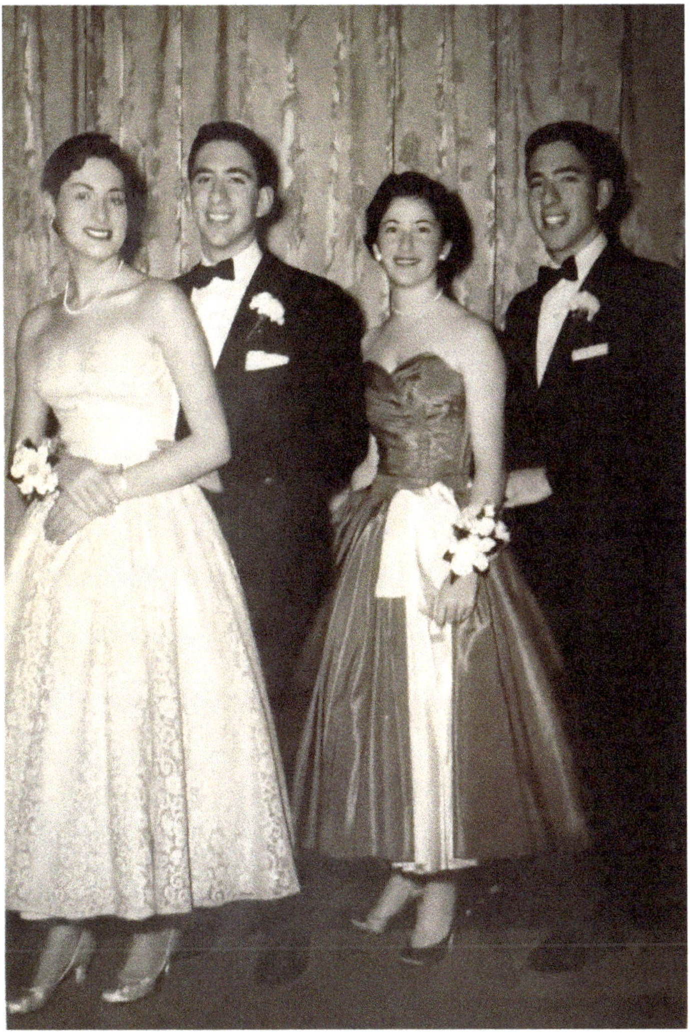

Stuart (left) and Jay at age 16 with their dates, Billi Goldberg and Elaine Toumarkine, for the senior prom in Wilmington, Delaware, 1956

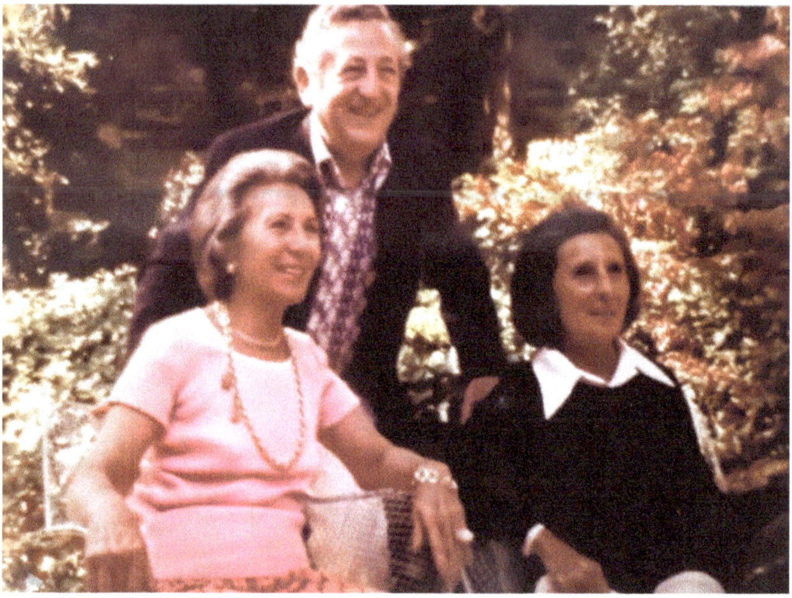

Ruth Levy (Jay's mother), her brother, Phil Blank, and their sister, Ann Young, at a family reunion in Philadelphia, 1955

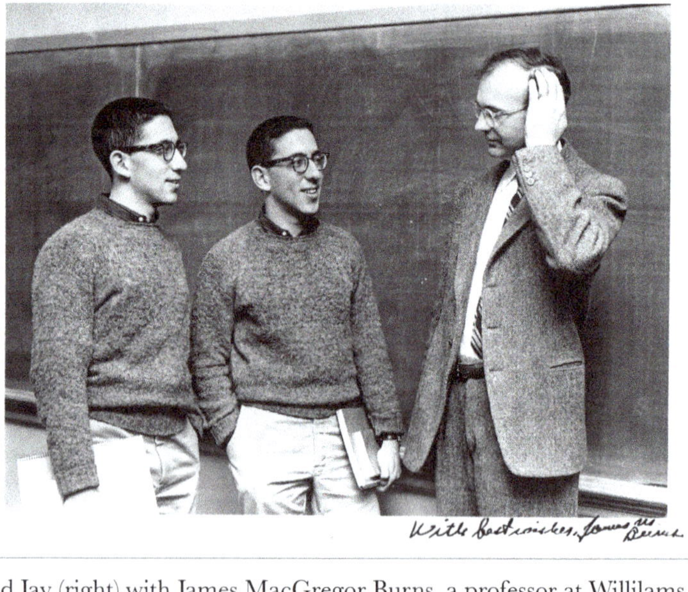

Stuart and Jay (right) with James MacGregor Burns, a professor at Willilams College, 1958. This photo was taken at the time of their switching colleges.

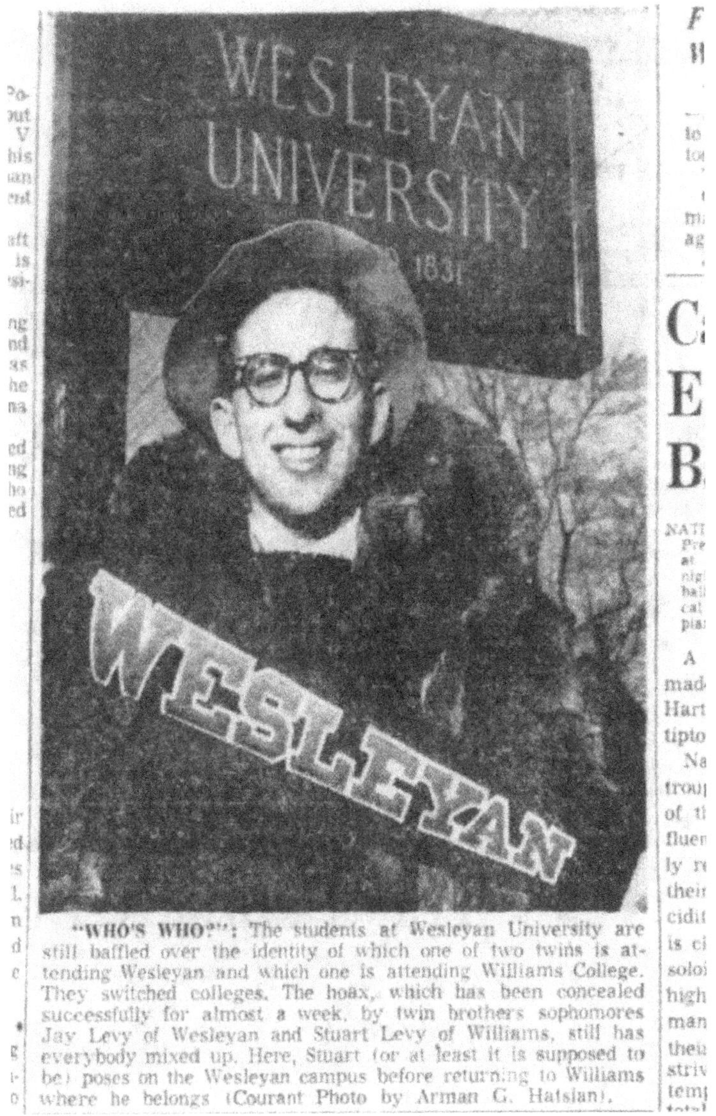

"WHO'S WHO?": The students at Wesleyan University are still baffled over the identity of which one of two twins is attending Wesleyan and which one is attending Williams College. They switched colleges. The hoax, which has been concealed successfully for almost a week, by twin brothers sophomores Jay Levy of Wesleyan and Stuart Levy of Williams, still has everybody mixed up. Here, Stuart (or at least it is supposed to be) poses on the Wesleyan campus before returning to Williams where he belongs (Courant Photo by Arman G. Hatsian).

Stuart in the *Hartford Courant* after he and Jay switched colleges for a week, 1958

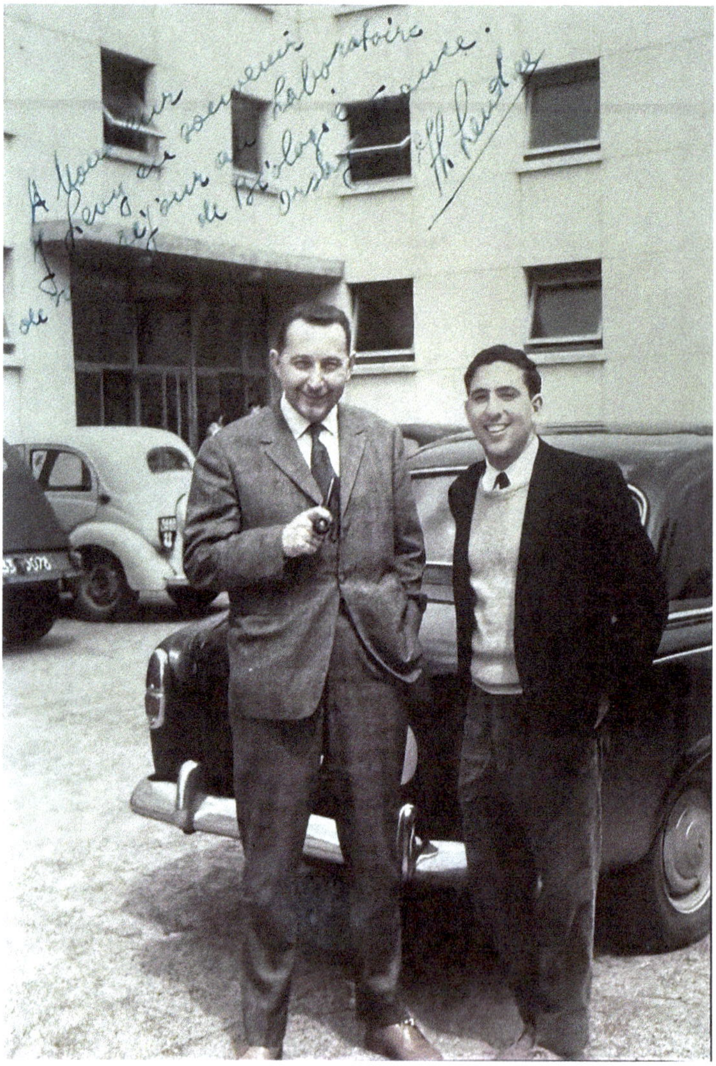

Jay with Tomas Lender, with whom he conducted research at the Faculty de Science in Orsay, France, 1960

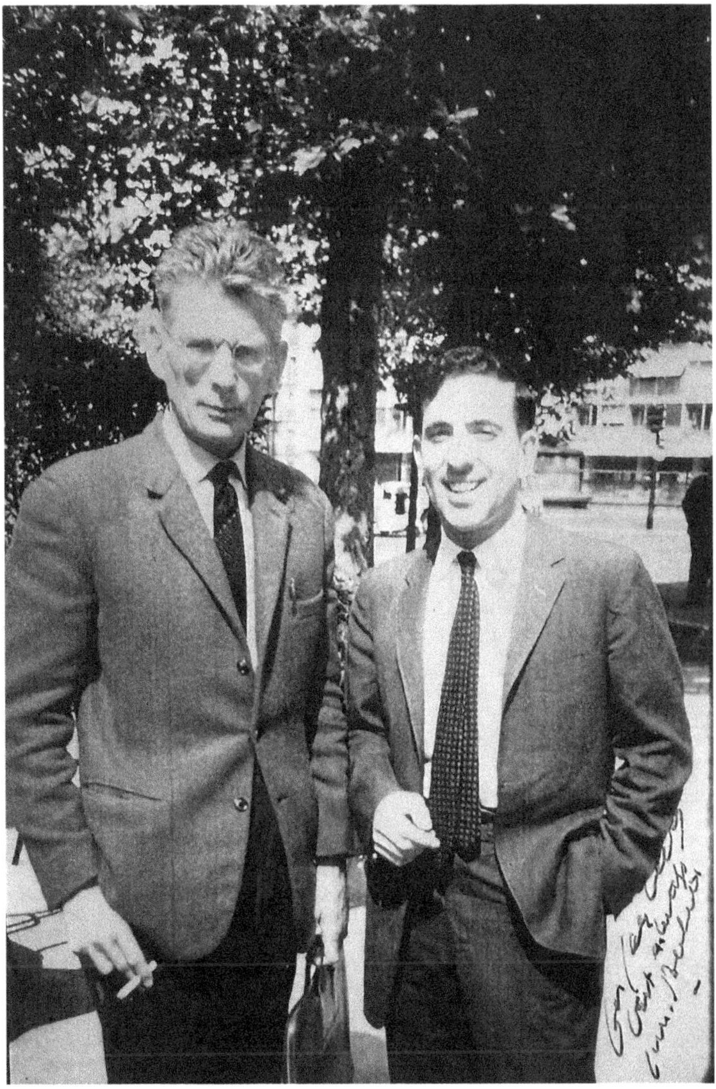

Jay's first meeting with Samuel Beckett in Paris, February 1961

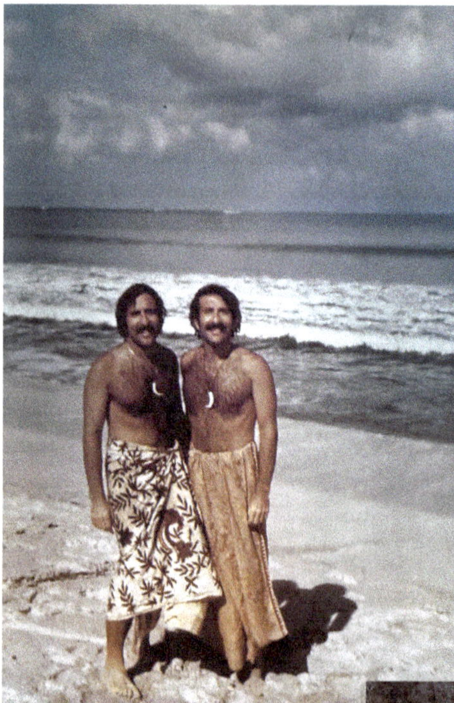

Jay (left) and Stuart in Bali, 1968

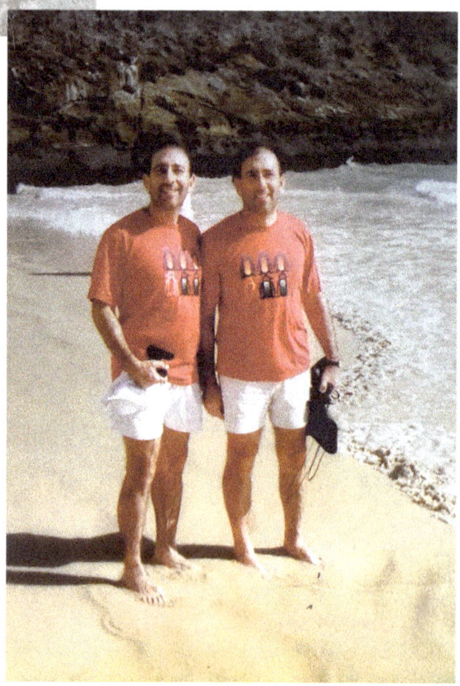

Stuart (left) and Jay in Bali, 1978

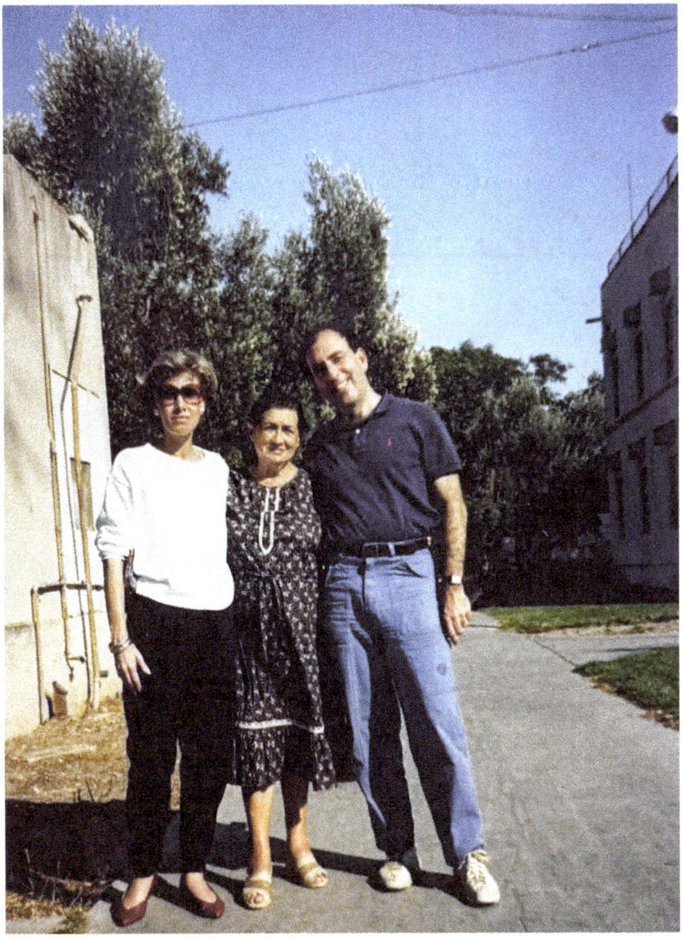

Sharon Levy, Panina Yeina, and Jay, Kibbutz Afikim in Israel, 1978

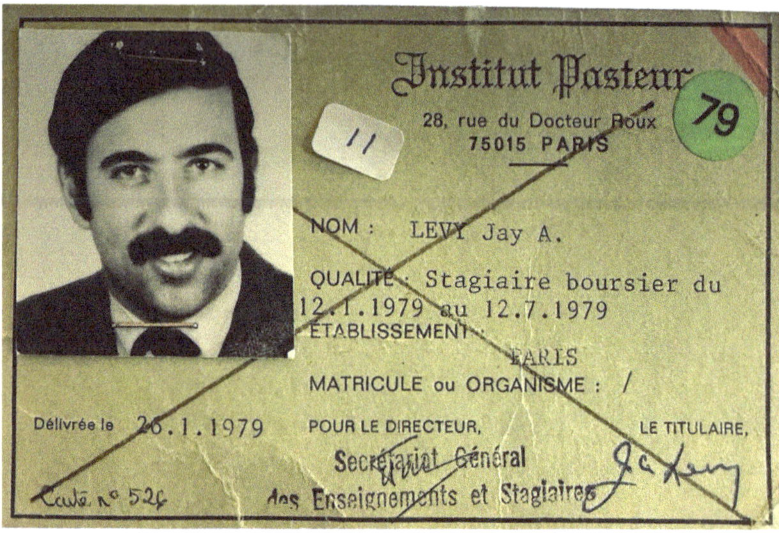

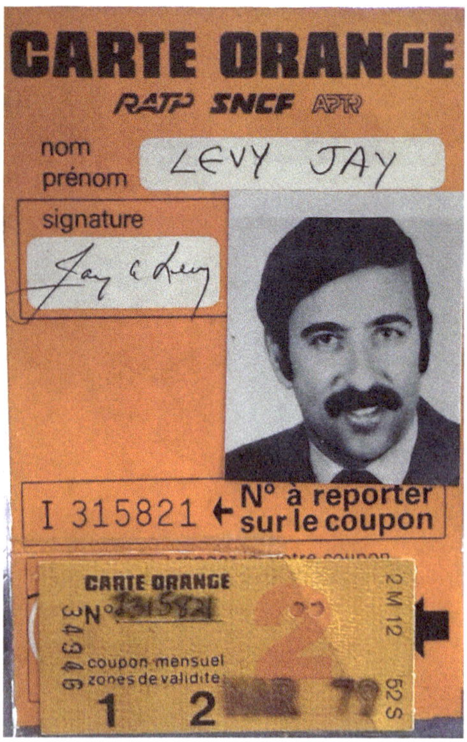

Jay's identity cards for the Pasteur Institute and for the Metro during his sabbatical in Paris, 1979

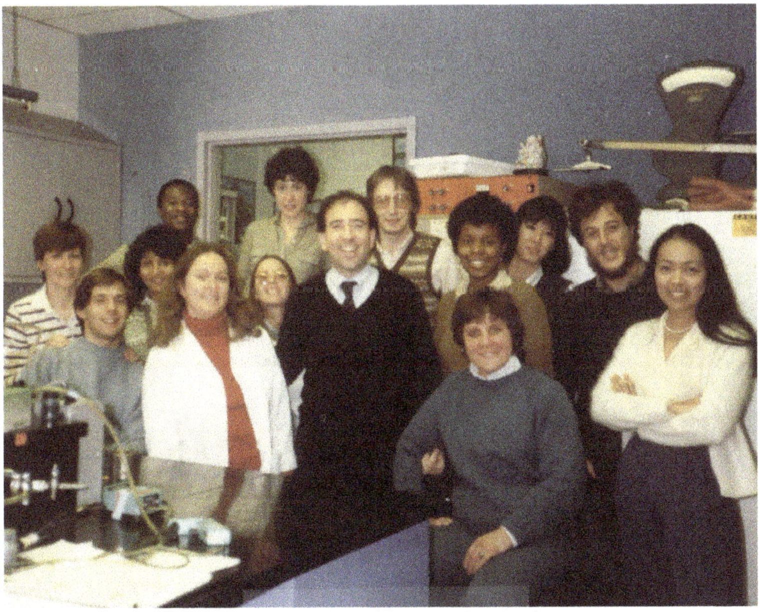

Jay's HIV/AIDS lab at UCSF, 1983

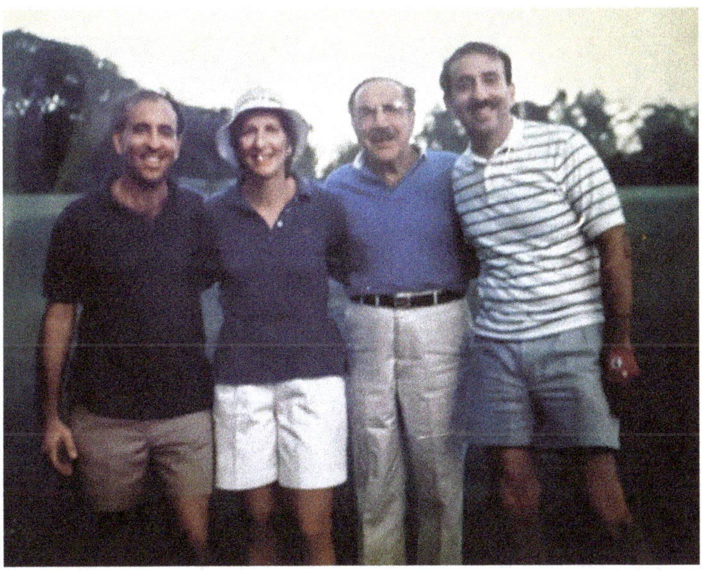

Jay (left) with his sister Ellen, brother Stuart, and their father Charles, in Williamsburg, Virginia, 1985

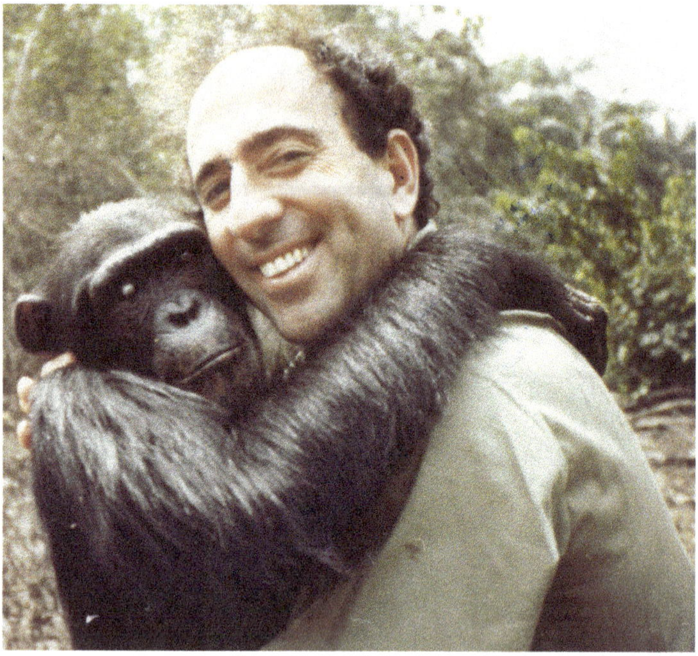

Jay's visit to a chimpanzee colony in the Ivory Coast, 1987

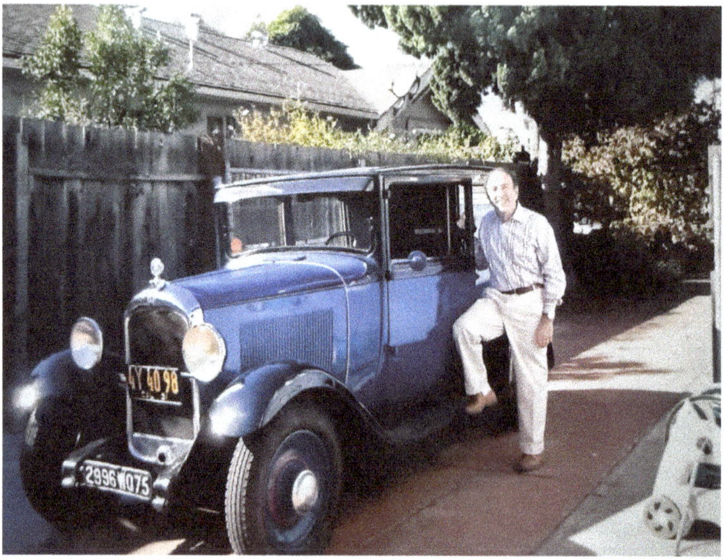

Jay with his antique C 4G Citroen car, 1993

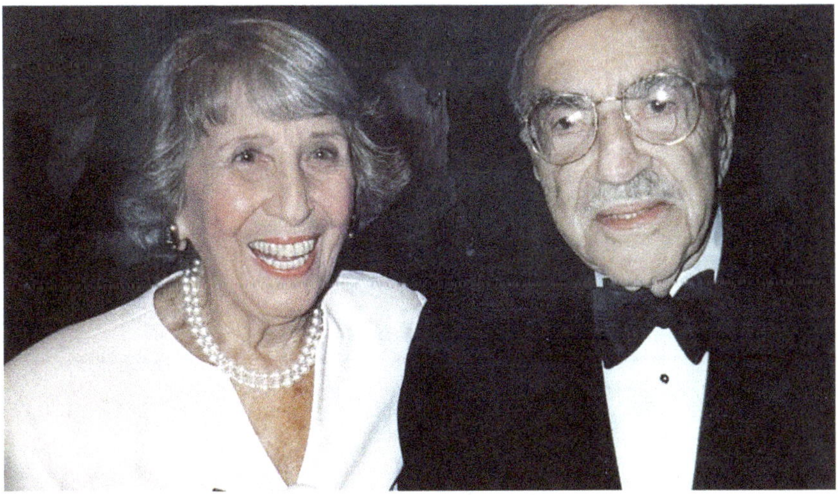

Jay's parents, Ruth and Charles Levy, 1993

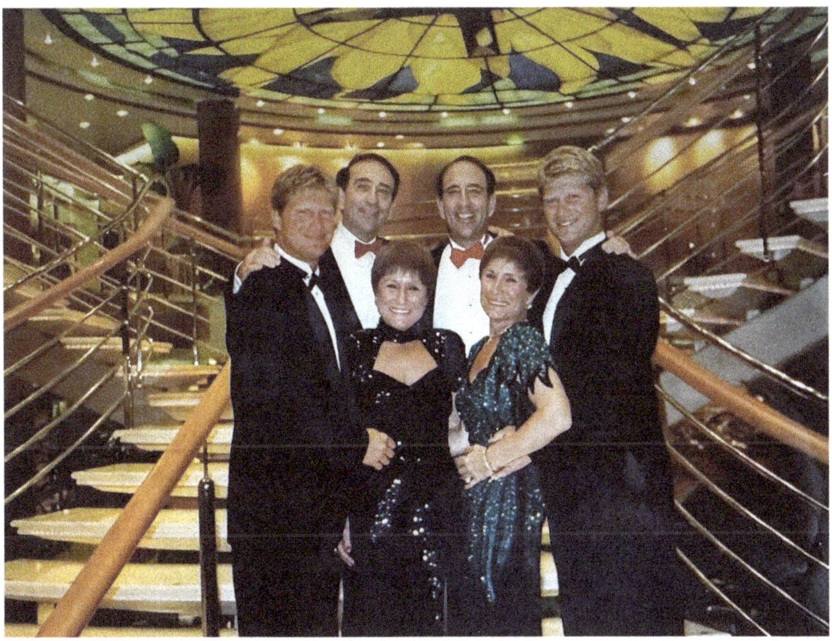

The Dawn Princess twins cruise, Stuart and Jay (right), Jimmy and Jerry McAlister, Lisa Goodwin and Gerda Kirkpatrick, 1996

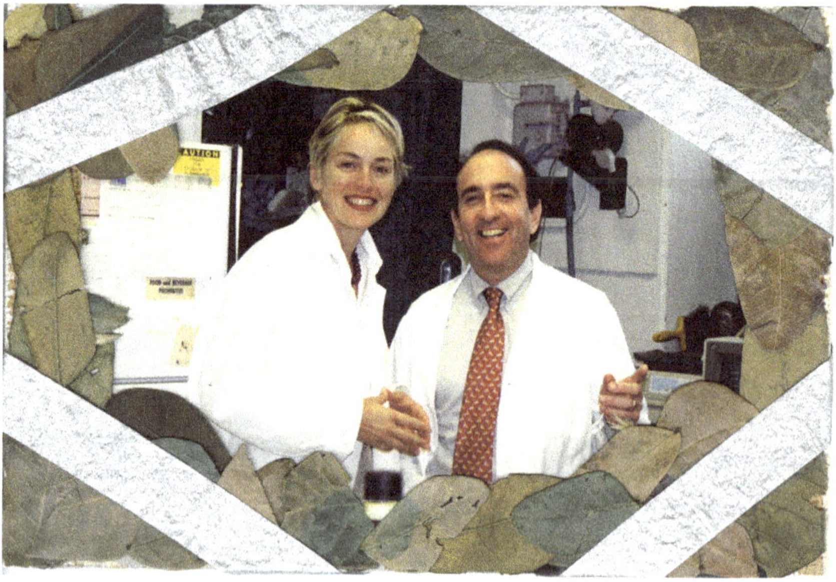

Jay with Sharon Stone on her visit to his UCSF lab, 1999

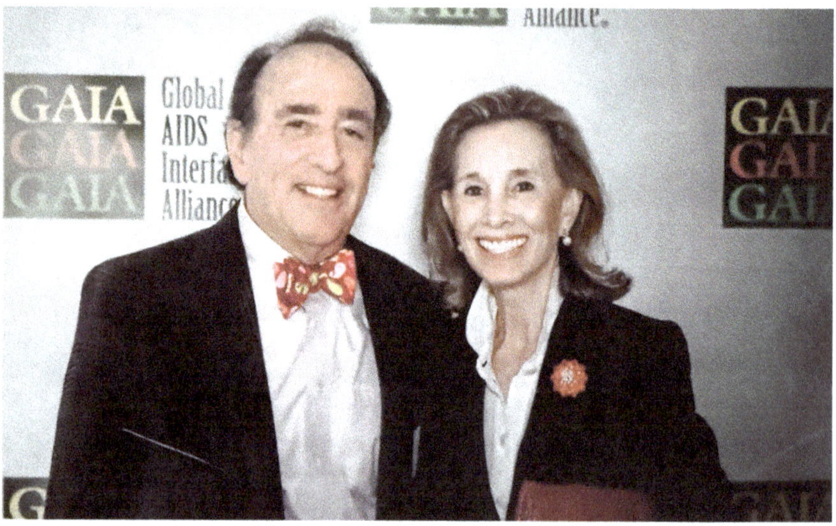

Jay and Sharon at an awards ceremony for the Global AIDS Interfaith Alliance (GAIA) in San Francisco, 2005

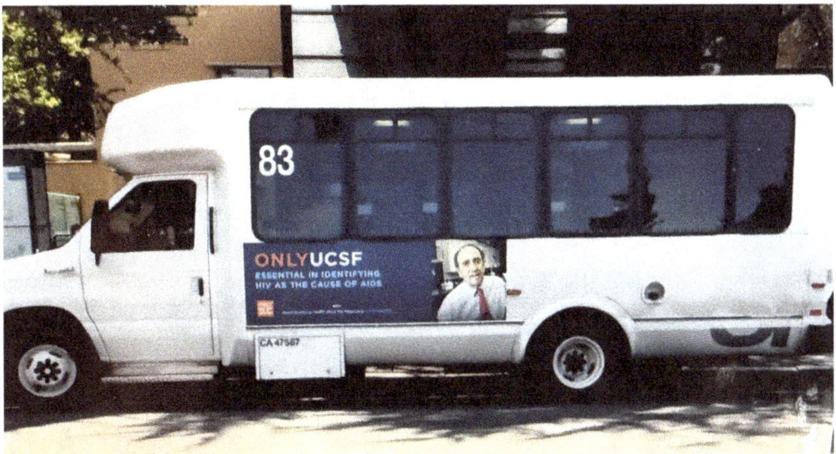

UCSF bus advertising Jay's research, 2011

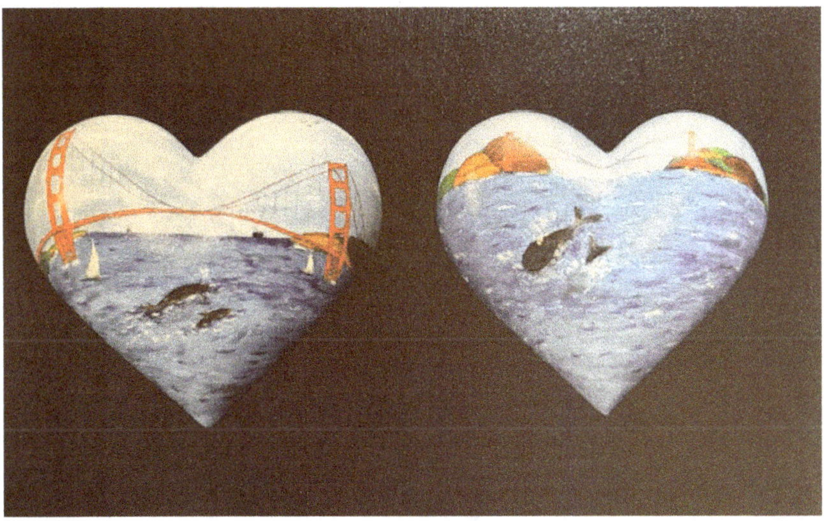

A ceramic heart painted on both sides by Jay which was purchased for $15,000 in an auction to benefit San Francisco General Hospital, 2014

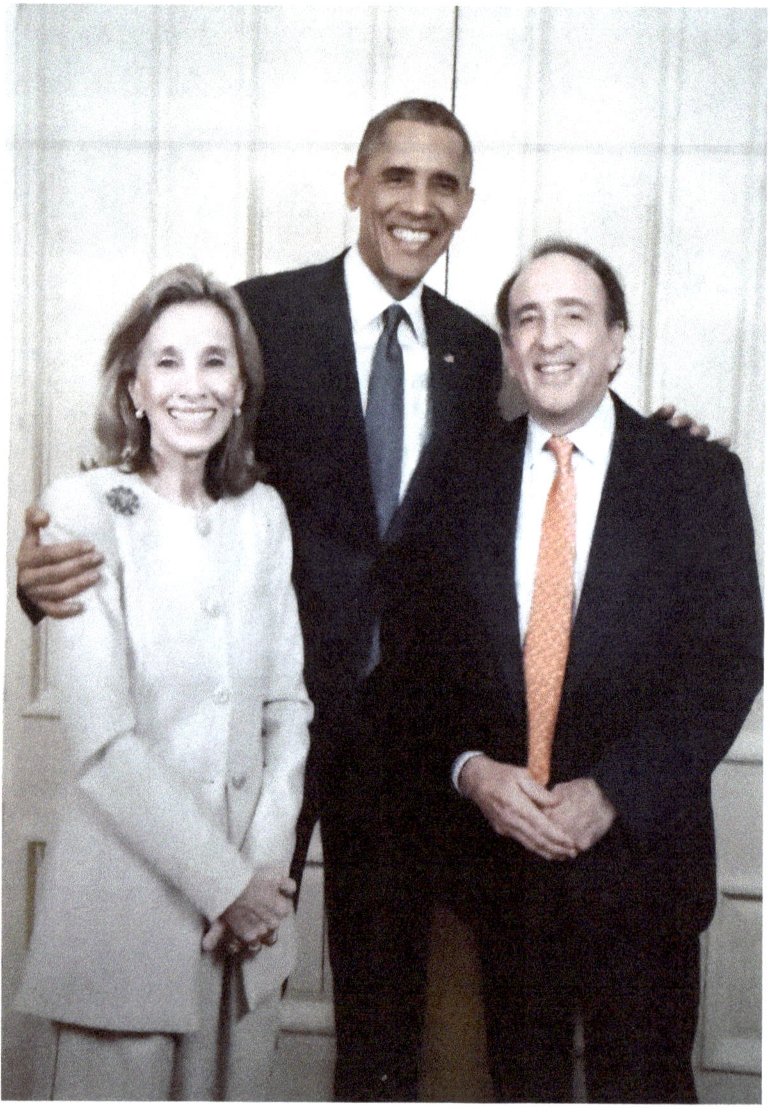

Sharon and Jay with President Barack Obama at a reception in San Francisco, 2013

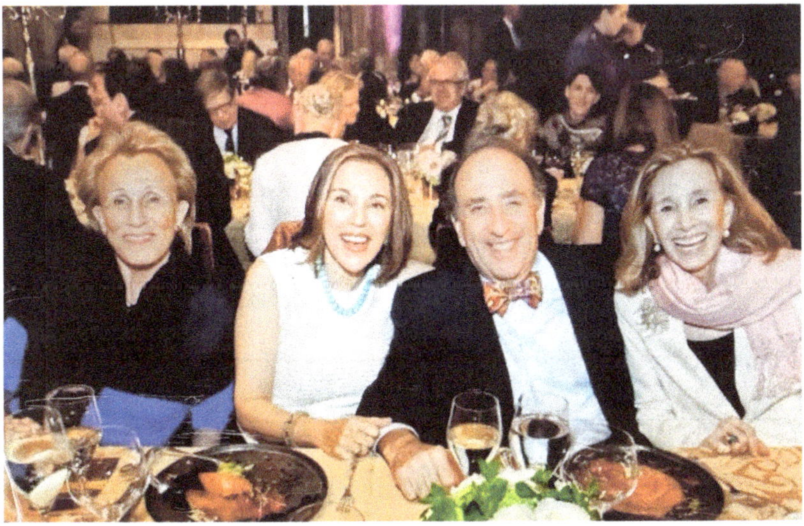

Jay with the "harem" that traveled with him on a cruise ship from Istanbul to Athens: Michele Michels, Laura Flug, Sharon, 2015

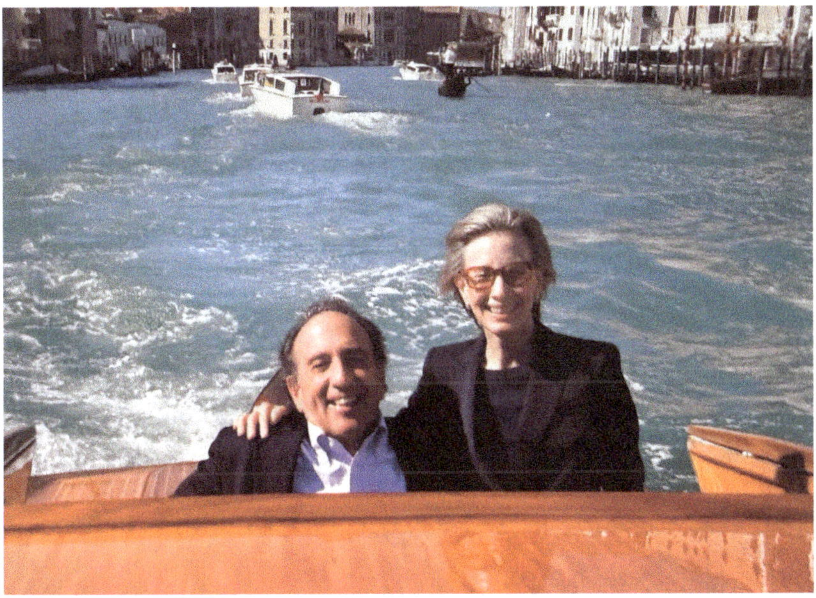

Jay and Sharon arriving in Venice by water taxi, 2018

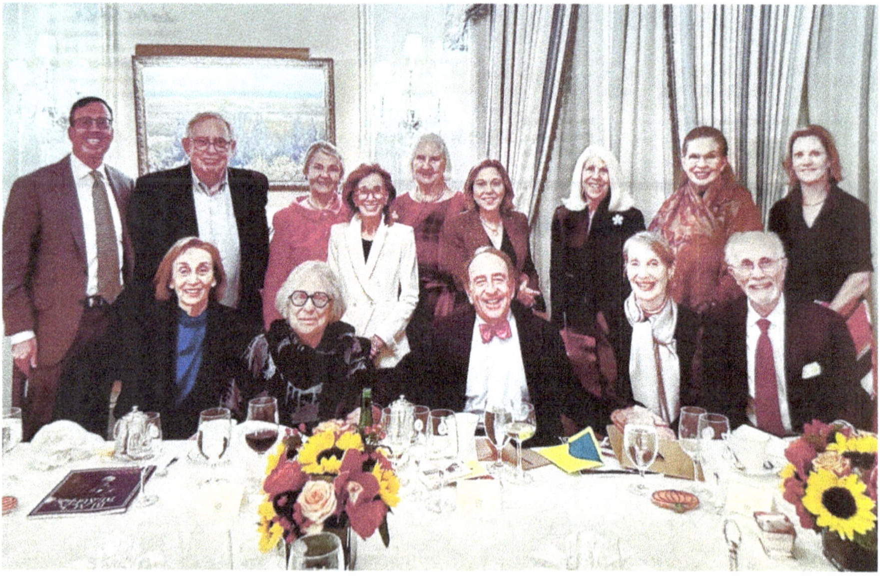

Jay's birthday party at the Lotos Club in New York, 2022
Back row: Matt Winn, Jack Blum, Anke Volcker, Sharon Levy, Liz Hylton, Laura Flug, Kandi Stroud, Paige Peterson, Sharon Winn
Front row: Toni Young, Liz Verville, Jay, Kathy Miller, David Miller

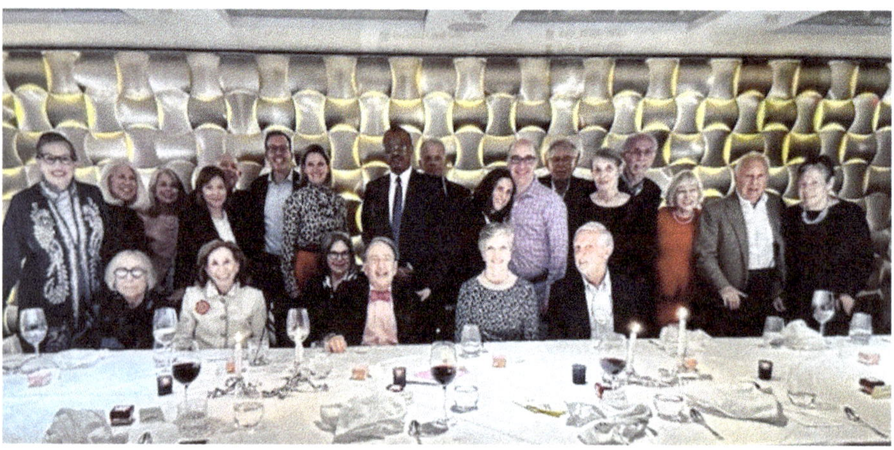

A group celebration of Jay's birthday at Café Milano in Washington, DC, 2023

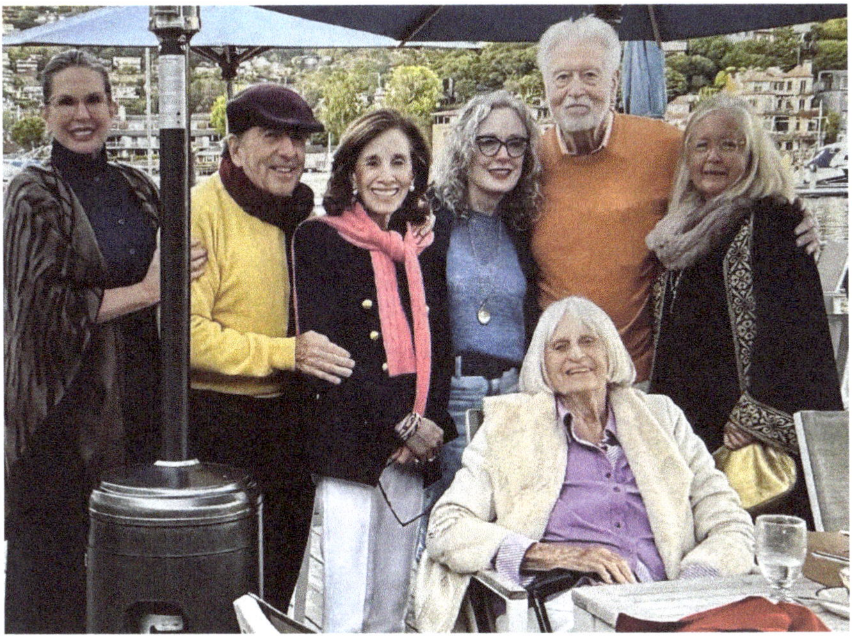

Saturday Covid pod lunch crew: Connie Wiley (seated); Paige Peterson, Jay, Sharon Levy, Cricket Jones, Rev. Alan Jones, Wendy Miller, 2023

Chapter 6

Going West, Starting Work, and Finding a Wife

After three years as a clinical associate at NIH, Jay was ready for a new challenge. Staying at NIH could have been an option and it would have carried cache. But it was still a government job and many of Jay's friends told him he shouldn't stay in the public sector.

He considered going back to New York, but one of his NIH colleagues, an immunologist named John Mills, suggested he go to California. "See what medicine is like on the West Coast," he told Jay, and encouraged him to apply to the University of California, San Francisco (UCSF) – a stand-alone medical school. Jay applied for a position there and other institutions, including Duke University. Duke's head of medicine, Jim Weingarden, had recently moved to Duke from Penn and he encouraged Jay to come there for a residency. But being young and single, Jay wasn't thrilled by the prospect of living alone in Durham, North Carolina. By contrast, "going to California seemed like a great idea," recalls Jay. "It was an adventure." San Francisco had been in the news for several years, because of anti-war protests and the emergence of hippies. (The fabled "summer of love" had been a few years earlier, in 1967.)

It was an unconventional choice. Unlike today, UCSF was not a top-tier medical school. No one else from Jay's class of clinical associates went there, given that the most prestigious medical schools were all on the east coast. But Jay liked the idea of going west and Mills convinced him it was the right choice. By contrast, Jay recalls that his parents were shocked. "They didn't know anyone in San Francisco. And they thought what many people thought – that the city had many crazy people."

When the offer arrived from UCSF, to start in 1970, Jay didn't hesitate to accept it. While others encouraged him to return to Penn, he felt his clinical skills needed improvement, so he continued his residency at UCSF, which gave him the opportunity to see patients who were in early stages of disease.

To prepare for the move, Jay bought a new Pontiac Firebird for about $3,500. It didn't take long for him to realize it was a lemon. During one outing, his girlfriend tried to close the passenger door, only to have the handle detach and end up in her hand.

When leaving Washington, DC for San Francisco, Jay didn't want to make the drive across the country on his own. He took out a classified ad in the *Washington Post,* saying he was looking for someone to join him and share the driving. A tall, long-haired 19-year-old student from California named Randy Small answered the ad. The two bonded quickly, and Jay set just one condition for the drive: if they were stopped by the police, Randy was not to exit the car.

The seven-day trip went off largely without a hitch – they did some camping along the way – though they were taken to a police station in Kansas for speeding and the car broke down once. Randy didn't get out of the car and the police did not make an issue of his bohemian appearance. While driving through Nevada, they were passing by an enclosure where they saw a young woman sunbathing in the nude. Curious, they pulled over. When they did, a few other fully nude individuals approached the car and invited them to go for a swim. They had unwittingly entered a nudist colony and ended up staying for a few days, with Jay and Randy enjoying their time in the buff.

Randy's family lived in Davis, California – a university town near

Sacramento – and when they were nearby, Randy asked to be dropped off near his house. His father, Arthur, was vice chancellor at UC Davis and they lived in a stately home, which Randy, as a hippie, may have found embarrassing. (Jay and Randy remained friends and Jay had 25 consecutive Thanksgiving dinners with the extended Small family during his time in San Francisco.)

When Jay finally arrived in San Francisco, he slept at the home of one of his Wesleyan classmates, Ken Hunter, who lived near the ocean. Jay spent his days and weekends looking for an apartment. He was drawn to Telegraph Hill, a largely residential area where many residences have sweeping views of the bay and the Bay Bridge.

While touring this neighborhood one weekend day, he struck up a conversation with a young woman named Joanie Levin, who was gardening in front of her home on the picturesque Napier Lane. She introduced Jay to her husband, Marvin, who quickly invited Jay on a driving tour of San Francisco and other nearby towns. They went over the Golden Gate Bridge to the waterfront community of Sausalito. But on their drive back, neither of them had money to pay the bridge toll to cross the Golden Gate Bridge and Marvin had to leave his wristwatch as collateral.

Meeting Joanie and Marvin was a *beshert* moment and convinced Jay that he wanted to live on Telegraph Hill. The Levins told him he needed to meet an influential local real estate agent, an 83-year-old woman named Grace Marchant, a former stunt woman who had grown up in South Dakota. Jay went to her antiquated home at the corner of the Filbert Street steps and Napier Lane and discovered she had about 12 cats. "I knew I needed to show some attention to her pets, so I let some of them sit on my lap during my hour-long talk with her," recalls Jay. She was taken by Jay, telling him the neighborhood needed a local doctor, though he later found out that her preferred remedy for any condition was a nip of turpentine. (She lived to be 96.)

About a week later, Jay was treating a patient in the clinic at UCSF when he received an urgent phone call. It was Marchant and she told Jay she had an apartment for him. He said he would come see it that weekend. She said he needed to come immediately: "you don't understand – it might not be available later." He had a colleague take over examining the patient and drove to the apartment, which was 134 steps up Telegraph Hill, at 231 Greenwich Street. "It was spacious and had a great view of the Bay Bridge," recalls Jay. "I immediately loved it."

Marchant had grown plants along the path to the apartment and one of them stood out, as Jay had never seen it before: Brugmansia, which is more commonly known as a trumpet flower or Datura and is derived from the potato family. In later years, the cultivation of this plant and its varieties would become a passion for Jay. At one time he had yellow, orange, red, white and double white flowering Daturas at his San Francisco home on Lake Street.

While the $250 monthly rent was steep for Jay – his salary was $750 per month – he signed the lease agreement. He remembered the popular advice that one's rent should be no more than one-third of one's salary. The apartment fit that advice very well.

Joanie and Marvin were thrilled to have Jay in the neighborhood and he had dinner with them every Thursday night. It marked the beginning of a friendship that lasted for 20 years. It only ended when Joanie's newborn child developed Tay-Sachs disease and she fell into depression. Joanie later moved to Pacifica and Marvin moved to Piedmont, with the result that Jay saw progressively less of each of them.

Jay recalls that his early years at UCSF were "pretty dull. I had a few girlfriends, but no one serious. I had a few other friends, some of whom were genuine and others who just wanted free medical advice. I talked to Stuart, who was living in Boston, almost every day. We had similar stories as we reminisced about our life as single men."

Given Jay's innate curiosity, he nonetheless liked living in a new place. And he experimented with what he calls San Francisco's "crazy stuff," which made the city the butt of many jokes throughout the country. He would often spend Thursday evenings after dinner with the Levins with friends in search of greater "meanings in life." The group sometimes practiced parapsychology (e.g., clairvoyance, ESP, telepathy), meditation, and visualization. He also attended a much-discussed self-improvement course known as "est," which was led by a motivational speaker named Werner Earhard.

Jay, at the time, was also reading a popular book that had been published in 1970, *Jonathan Livingston Seagull*. Written by Richard Bach as an allegorical fable, it contained ideas that Jay would later be drawn to in *The Celestine Prophecy*. A key idea in the book – a bird's quest to fly higher – became the motto of Jay's lab ("reach higher heights"). He cites the book as the reason why he petitioned UCSF (successfully) to change the paint color on the walls of his renovated lab rooms from yellow and green to mauve and royal blue. (Yellow and green were widely-used for industrial colors at the time.) As earth colors, it was expected they would bring energy and an innovation to the rooms. Jay thought otherwise.

"I liked all of this because it was a brand new experience for me and it was so far outside science," recalls Jay. "I thought then, and think now, that it's important for researchers to balance their scientific absolutism with an appreciation for what can seem magical or mystical. And these experiences were what opened me to other *beshert* experiences."

Throughout this time, Jay was still involved with clinical work and took pride in intervening during a woman's difficult pregnancy and getting an attending physician to tend to her – helping to save the woman's life. (She was the wife of Norman Myers, a celebrated nature photographer from England; they were vacationing in San Francisco.) But he had no long-term plan and expected to return to the east coast after his residency concluded.

It's Greek to me

During his medical Residency at Penn, Jay would sometimes go to a Philadelphia bar called Tip Top that served Greek food. The experience left Jay feeling a strong kinship with Greek people. "I think in my former life I was a Greek sailor," says Jay. "But I have no idea why."

When Jay arrived in San Francisco, he asked colleagues where he could find authentic Greek food. Living in Philadelphia during his residency he learned Greek music and dancing. He was also directed to a restaurant on Eddy Street in the Tenderloin – then (and now) a shady part of San Francisco – and it had a distinctly un-Greek name: The Golden Peacock.

On Jay's first visit, he struck up a conversation with the waiter, Peter Stavros, who was the son of the owner. Peter introduced his mother, Stella, to Jay, and they had an immediate connection: she spoke Yiddish, having grown up in Salonika, a large city in Greece that had once been home to a large Jewish population.

"The restaurant became my home away from home," recalls Jay, and not just because he could get a dinner of lemon soup and grape leaves for $1.50. The Stavros family adopted Jay and he became close friends with their daughter, Yvoni – so much so that he served as her best man (*koumbaros*) at her wedding. "I was welcomed into the San Francisco Greek community" says Jay, who was so fond of Greek gatherings that over the years he would go to one of their restaurants, Salonika, when it was hosting a Greek wedding reception. (If anyone asked, he would say he was a close friend of the caterer.) Jay learned about Greek dancing and Greek cuisine from Peter and Yvoni and participated in several family gatherings. Jay and Sharon remain friendly with the family – the children call him *"theios,"* which is Greek for "uncle." "We invited them to special occasions and they did the same for us" says Jay. That family connection continues today.

Sharon

One of the major examples of *beshert* in Jay's life was the way in which he met the woman who would become his wife. Jay had stayed in contact with the Small family and Arthur, the father and the vice chancellor at UC-Davis would sometimes call Jay seeking medical advice. Also, Arthur and his wife, Marion, would sometimes stay in Jay's Telegraph Hill apartment when he was away.

One day in early 1977, Arthur called Jay to ask him to meet a student of his at UC Davis. The student, Andy Kluger, was helping find lodging for Russian Jewish women who were being settled in San Francisco. Arthur wanted Jay to give Kluger some advice on living in the city. Jay agreed to the meeting and he brought a Russian woman from his lab, Oksana. At the end of one session, Kluger asked Jay to meet again, but this time at a local place on Broadway, to help prostitutes resolve their legal problems. Kluger wore a raincoat that reminded Jay of a character Peter Falk played in the popular TV show, "Columbo."

It was all a bit bizarre, recalls Jay, but a few weeks after they had met, Kluger mentioned that he had recently met a girl at a dinner party and recommended that Jay call her for a date. Kluger called Jay twice to remind him to make the call. Jay was intrigued, so he called the woman, Sharon Gulkus. They arranged to meet late one Sunday afternoon at a party near the woman's apartment in Sausalito. It was on the basement level of the Casa Madrona Hotel in Sausalito. "I had been on several blind dates," recalls Jay, "and I didn't expect this one to be any different." In fact, he arrived late because he he'd just been on a date with a woman from Burlingame.

It was a crowded party, so Jay and Sharon sat on a couch and talked. "I was impressed," recalls Jay. "Sharon reminded me of attractive co-eds I had met at University of Pennsylvania, including my cousin Ronell Young, who lived in Philadelphia with her husband Bill Douglass." Jay and Sharon also had many things in common, including frequent gatherings of their extended families on weekends and having grown up not far from each other (Sharon was from Philadelphia, which can be only about 30 minutes by car from Wilmington). When Jay bid her goodbye at the end of that first evening, he said he would contact her after returning from Santo Domingo, where he was going for the Christmas holidays to visit his sister, Ellen. It was two weeks before he called. Sharon thought he said "San Diego" and wondered why it took so long for him to call.

When Jay came to pick her up for one of their dates, and waited in her Sausalito apartment for her to get ready, her radio was playing the Elvis Presley ballad, "Can't Help Falling in Love." That became their special song.

Not long before meeting Jay, Sharon had consulted a fortune teller/ palm reader named Maris, who was said to have taught at Stanford. She predicted that Sharon would meet a man during the Christmas season who would have a close family like hers from the east coast and that they would marry by the time of her birthday, in July. It didn't take long for Jay to be smitten with Sharon, and when he sent her a Valentine's card about six weeks after their first date, he told a friend, "I'm sending this card to the woman I am going to marry."

Their dates included ski trips and golfing outings. "Sharon participated but did not show great talent," recalls Jay. She was also on a diet when they were dating and he joked that he could take her to expensive restaurants to impress her, since she wouldn't eat very much. She understood that Jay had a busy schedule and during their courtship, he recalls, "she never complained if I had to break a date."

Six months after Jay and Sharon had met, they spent a night in the Mendocino Lodge in northern Marin County. He read her a poem he composed professing his love for her (he had written others for her, as was the tradition in his family for special occasions) and then popped the question. It took Sharon by surprise, but she was elated.

The next morning, Jay called Sharon's mother in Philadelphia to ask for Sharon's hand in marriage (Sharon's father had passed away). Her mother's amusing reply – "that is so wonderful; you know she's worth $1 million!" – was repeated at family gatherings for many years.

A Philadelphia wedding and Papua New Guinea honeymoon

They didn't want to wait long to get married and set a date of September 1, 1977, at the Barclay Hotel in Philadelphia. They chose that weekend thinking the weather would be hospitable, but it turned out to be an extremely hot day.

For the wedding, Sharon wore an apricot-colored dress and Jay wore a brown suit, though in retrospect, neither liked what they wore. Jay and his brother Stuart walked down the aisle together (Stuart, dressed as Jay's twin, was the best man). About 75 people attended – in addition to the usual family members and close friends, Jay's mentors from Wesleyan and NIH were also there. It was a traditional Jewish wedding ceremony, conducted by the same rabbi who had married Jay's parents in Wilmington. It ended with the traditional gesture of the groom using his foot to break a glass, which commemorates the challenges and destruction faced by Jews for thousands of years. (Jay was nervous about stepping on a drinking glass, so he used a lightbulb.)

The party went until about 11 p.m. (Jay's mother told him at 10:30 that the attendees were waiting for Jay and Sharon to declare the event over). The only drama came when Sharon's brother, Steve, coming down the steps, dropped the slice of wedding cake that was supposed to be saved for Jay and Sharon's one-year anniversary.

The next day, Jay and Sharon were flying from Philadelphia to San Francisco. At the airport, Jay realized that he had left his suits and sport coats in their room at the Barclay Hotel. He had them delivered to the airport by taxi. After a brief stay in San Francisco, they flew to Hawaii to relax for a few days before going on to Japan, where Jay was speaking at a cancer meeting. Stuart was with Jay and Sharon for these early days of their honeymoon as he was also speaking at the same cancer meeting.

Sharon had wanted to go to Africa for the honeymoon. But Jay had already been there and hoped to go somewhere he hadn't been previously. They settled on another exotic location: Papua New Guinea, which was known for kuru, a disease caused by a replicating protein, a prion. They were booked on a river boat down the Sepik River, which is the longest river in the country. It was not a luxury outing. They slept on the boat and there was little protection from mosquitoes, which resulted in Sharon getting at least 20 bites on one of her toes.

When they woke up after the first night on the river raft, Jay encountered a local young man playing a guitar and wearing a Boston Red Sox jersey. "I was worried," recalls Jay. "The village seemed to have been overrun with tourists and I wanted Sharon to have an experience akin to the ones I had in Africa, with natives in tribal clothes." His fears were all for naught. He and Sharon spent seven days touring, with four other travelers on the boat with them (another couple and two women from Australia). They rarely encountered other tourists. The group didn't cross paths with any of the country's tribes that still practiced cannibalism, but Jay and Sharon still didn't always feel safe.

When the boat tour ended, they were let off in a small village. They were scheduled to stay overnight in a hotel and then be driven to an airport in Wewak – the capital of a province in New Guinea – to fly to Australia. They were told to meet their driver at a local bar, but the driver didn't show. As Jay and Sharon waited, they started to be harassed by locals, who accused them of making off with local art works. Two local boys who were about nine years old approached Jay and Sharon and offered to help. Unsure of what to do, Jay accepted their offer – and left Sharon outside the bar with one of the boys. (Jay learned from his time in Africa that when faced with a predicament, planning for an exit should be the top priority.)

Jay proceeded to walk for about a half mile with the other boy into the forest. They arrived at the residence of the boys' boss – a tall, thin Australian man, about 35 years old, who was wearing a Speedo-style bikini bathing suit and who managed the plantation where the boys' father worked. The man happened to be wearing a necklace adorned with a large Star of David. (He was not Jewish – the necklace was a gift from his girlfriend.) Jay recognized this as a *beshert* moment and murmured to himself, "Our prayers have been answered." The man said he would drive Jay in his truck and return to the bar to pick up Sharon and then drive them to the airport, though he insisted on finishing his dinner first. Jay recalls,

> He seemed annoyed at being interrupted and was not very sympathetic to our situation. He was probably accustomed to these episodes. The truck was fairly old but I was relieved to see it. The driver had to negotiate rocky dirt roads and as we approached the bar, he told me the truck had no brakes and that I needed to drag my feet outside to help slow us down. Fortunately, he drove slowly. It was a great relief for Sharon when we arrived, as I had been gone for about 45 minutes. She got into the truck and was remarkably calm during this sudden adventure. When we were several miles from the airport, I noticed that the gas gauge was on empty. The driver replied casually, "Yeah, sometimes it doesn't work." The experience was so stressful, I got a severe stomach pain, like an ulcer. But we made it to Wewak, where we had to spend the night in a hotel before catching our flight to Darwin, Australia. It was very disquieting!

The next morning at the airport, the airline's representatives told Jay and Sharon they were not on the passenger manifest and would have to wait for the next flight, which was five days later. Panicking, Jay grabbed the passenger manifest, pointed at two random names and said, "that's us." The airline reps never bothered to check and let them board the plane.

Another adventure unfolded when they tried to change traveler's checks at their hotel in Darwin. They were told they'd need to do this at a local bank. Upon returning from the bank, the staff apologized for the inconvenience of obtaining money, saying that they refused their request because Jay and Sharon resembled a couple that was wanted for robbing banks – a young man with a mustache and his blonde wife. "Ironically, I had been sporting a mustache for at least a year," recalls Jay, "and I had promised Sharon I would shave it off during this trip. We agreed it would be the night in Darwin. We laughed thinking the staff would consider the change in my look was in response to the robbery inquiry."

While in Darwin, Jay visited an Aboriginal village and gave a lecture about hygiene. But it was very hot in the hut where he was scheduled to speak, and the stench so strong, that he spoke from the doorway, while everyone in attendance remained inside.

Soon thereafter, Jay and Sharon then flew to Sydney, where they saw friends, followed by a visit to Tahiti, where they had a cabin on a small island for a few days, and then flew home – having been on the road for over five weeks. "We were thrilled with the excitement and diversity of our adventures," recalls Jay.

Starting out in San Francisco

When they returned from the honeymoon, Sharon moved into Jay's Greenwich Street apartment, but she wasn't enamored with navigating the neighborhood's 134 steps and they agreed to look for a house in another neighborhood. A friend recommended Lake Street in the Richmond district, adjacent to the Presidio. Their plan was to rent, but they saw a sign for a house that was for sale on Lake Street, by 12th Avenue. It was owned by a doctor, and when they went to see it, the owner told Jay he could hire him as a medical consultant on issues around asbestos exposure and mesothelioma. Both Jay and Sharon liked the house, so they sought advice from Jay's best friend in San Francisco, Norman Buckhardt, who knew real estate in the Bay Area. He said the house wasn't worth the asking price of $179,000 but that they "should buy it anyway," saying that real estate in San Francisco could be trusted to appreciate in value. It was good advice. "After several decades of ownership," says Jay, "it is our most valuable asset."

Jay and Sharon offered the full asking price at the recommendation of friends of theirs who were real estate agents, Rick and JoAnn Soued. Another friend of Jay and Sharon who regularly bought and sold homes in San Francisco visited the house. He was adamant they shouldn't buy it. Sharon's mother also visited some weeks later and was appalled that the house had no closets. And while houses were in high demand, Jay refused to increase the bid. To his wonderful surprise, the seller accepted their offer. And it's still the house Jay and Sharon live in today. Another *beshert.*

Chapter 7

Diagnosing an Epidemic Amid Institutional Resistance

On August 6, 1981, Jay was in room S 1280 of the Medical Sciences building on UC San Francisco's Parnassus Avenue campus when he received a phone call from Paul Volberding, a young physician who was the head of oncology at San Francisco General Hospital. Volberding was doing his post-medical training in hematology and oncology at UCSF, which he had chosen because he wanted to conduct research with Jay.

"We have a young man with Kaposi's sarcoma (KS)," Volberding said to Jay. "With your known interest in cancer viruses, we would like you to come to the hospital's Medical Grand Rounds and give a talk on the possible cause of this disease." Volberding, who had spent the previous two years as Jay's research associate, studying mouse retroviruses and cancer, went on to say that while KS was very unusual in young men, rising numbers of them were afflicted with this cancer, particularly gay men: "It could be caused by an infectious agent!"

The gathering at SFGH four days after Volberding's call featured a presentation by a hematology fellow, Donald Abrams. It focused on the KS case and the possible role of a herpes virus in this cancer. Following Abrams' presentation, Jay said it was possible that the herpes viruses could cause this tumor, though he expressed surprise that the virus particles were seen by electron microscopy in the tumor itself.

Jay noted that if a virus transforms a cell, it typically remains latent in that cell and produces proteins that transform the cell into a malignant phenotype. The virus itself does not form an infectious particle. The biologic process transforms the cell but the virus, not fully formed, does not have the ability to replicate and kill the cell. "I said that the herpesviruses could be infecting this tumor and not be directly responsible for the cancer," recalls Jay, who had seen several cases of KS during his time in Uganda. (Several years later, a new herpesvirus was found associated with KS.[20])

This was Jay's introduction to what was known at the time as the "Gay Related Immune Deficiency" syndrome, or GRID. KS was a common cancer in patients with GRID as well as lymphomas – both of which were connected to a disorder in the immune system of the KS patients. That disorder, which in 1982 would be rechristened "Acquired Immune Deficiency Syndrome," or AIDS, clinically resembled the flu with myalgias and other observed symptoms common in viral infections. Afflicted individuals experienced muscle aches and fatigue and could have symptoms of neurologic disease. This syndrome was later found by Jay and others to be caused by a new human retrovirus, which was labeled the "human immunodeficiency virus" or HIV.

In the years that followed, millions of people would die of AIDS, in the United States and throughout the world. But helplessness gradually turned to hope, following the development of a treatment known as antiretroviral therapy (ART).[21] This therapy has been transformative. While AIDS was once a death sentence, today it's a treatable condition and people with HIV are more likely to die of other causes. As of 2016, the age-adjusted HIV death rate in the United States was more than 80 percent lower than it had been in 1995.[22] Globally, the number of AIDS-related deaths has declined by 70 percent since peaking in 2004 and by 54 percent since 2010.[23] "The response to AIDS will be a benchmark against which responses to future health threats will be compared," according to a paper written by researchers at the CDC and Emory University.[24]

Jay was at the forefront of this progress, having co-discovered the link between HIV and AIDS. This scientific breakthrough had far-reaching health implications. As Anthony Fauci has written,

> This advance led to the development of diagnostic assays that provided, for the first time, insight into the true scope of the outbreak. It became clear that patients presenting with advanced disease were just the tip of the iceberg and that orders of magnitude more people globally were living with HIV infection but had not yet developed obvious clinical disease. Building on these initial studies, researchers studying the epidemiology and natural history of HIV provided a snapshot of the full scope of a global epidemic.[25]

Jay's other breakthrough achievements included being the first to: clone the HIV genome, demonstrate how heat treatment could kill HIV in clotting factors (which protected many hemophiliacs from AIDS), report HIV in genital fluids and the brain, and show how cells of the immune system control HIV replication.

When Luc Montagnier, a French scientist, was awarded the Nobel Prize in 2008 for having discovered HIV, he singled out Jay's research for having "confirmed and extended" his findings.[26]

Early research and funding challenges

In August 1981, at the time Jay spoke at San Francisco General Hospital, much remained unknown about AIDS. Just two months earlier, the CDC had published a report about five gay men who had died of a rare form of pneumonia. The report's authors characterized this as "unusual," since none of them had a known underlying immunodeficiency.[27]

In the months that followed, the condition began to attract more attention. In May 1982, the CDC published another report on AIDS, saying it had afflicted 335 people – 136 of whom had already died. A *New York Times* article on the report – headlined "New Homosexual Disorder Worries Health Officials" – quoted the head of the National Cancer Institute, Bruce Chabner, who said AIDS was "of concern to all Americans."[28]

As the magnitude of the AIDS threat came into focus, Jay said to a doctor friend of his, "I have to find the cause of this disease." He recalled later, "It was in my mind that I was almost uniquely positioned to meet this challenge, given my international experience, particularly in Africa, and my background in virology, especially my recent work on retroviruses, coupled with the fact that I lived in a city that was being devastated by AIDS. The challenge, which was to find the causative agent, was a *beshert* moment for me."

What exactly is a retrovirus? The Cleveland Clinic offers a useful explanation:

> A retrovirus is a virus that works backward from the way human cells do. Human cells have instructions (DNA) that send a message (RNA) to make building blocks for your body (proteins). Retroviruses have their instructions written on RNA. When a retrovirus invades your cells, it changes its RNA to look like your cells' instructions (DNA). Then it cuts your cells' DNA and inserts its instructions into them. Your cell then acts as though the virus' instructions are its own.

HIV, points out the Cleveland Clinic, is a retrovirus. "All viruses invade your cells and then use your cells' 'machinery' to make more copies of themselves. HIV not only uses your cells to make more of itself, but it also inserts its instructions into your DNA."[29]

During the early days of Jay's research, he was introduced to a patient with KS and wanted to study it and try to isolate a possible causative virus. But there was an obstacle: the biosafety hood he was using for mouse work at UCSF did not meet the safety standard for infectious human virus work. He needed $1,500 (about $5,300 today) to purchase a filter for the hood.

But he encountered multiple obstacles while trying to secure the money. The Reagan Administration had slashed federal funding for medical research. These cutbacks led to all of Jay's grant proposals being dismissed. In 1981, his lab shrank to four people and UCSF's dean, Rudi Schmid, wrote to Jay and said if he (Jay) could not secure grant funding within a year, he would be terminated. The threat was a surprise for Jay, given that he had attracted grants of several hundred thousand dollars for virologic research.

"With all the obstacles in my way, I considered writing a novel about the endogenous inherited retroviruses, teaching at high schools or colleges or participating in a TV program to which I was invited by the *Journal of the American Medical Association* (JAMA) to explain medicine to the public," recalls Jay. "That was very attractive since I enjoyed teaching and I thought I could be the Carl Sagan of the biomedical field."

He secured a $35,000 grant from the National Science Foundation, to examine whether retroviruses would prevent the normal differentiation of the cells, which helped him get through this period. And one of his former NIH colleagues, Frank Rauscher, helped him secure a $50,000 grant from the American Cancer Society

But when Jay requested funding from the UCSF Chancellor, Julius

"Julie" Krevans, for the biosafety hood filter, Krevans told him there was no money available for it and recommended that he apply for a REAC (Research Evaluation Allocations Committee) grant for the funding. When Jay replied that it would take at least nine months to obtain those funds, and that there was an urgent health need to get started right away, Krevans held firm and said he could not find the funds.

Jay shared this story with a UCSF dermatologist, Marcus Conant, who replied that he had some connections in the state legislature. Six weeks later, Jay had the money. Soon thereafter, Jay was summoned to meet with Schmid, the UCSF dean, who asked him, "Why did you go around my back to get this money?" Jay later wrote that, "I left the Dean's office thinking I am relieved that I can work but I feel now the space that will be needed to do the research probably will not be given to me by the Dean."[30]

As Jay conducted his AIDS research, he also needed $50,000 to purchase an ultra-centrifuge that would enable him to concentrate fluids from cultured cells of AIDS patients to look for a causative agent. He asked Krevans about securing the funds but got nowhere.

There was another option. In May 1983, Jay was one of six researchers from academic medical centers in Northern California invited to meet with the speaker of the State Assembly, Willie Brown. Brown represented San Francisco and wanted to tackle the disease that was ravaging many of his constituents. To that end, he was going to submit an AIDS appropriation bill to the legislature.

When they arrived at Brown's Los Angeles office very early in the morning, Brown had six secretaries on hand to begin working on the appropriations bill. Jay's memories included Brown's fluorescent green tie – he was well known for being a sharp dresser – and that the secretaries had what was at the time cutting-edge technology: self-correcting typewriters.

The group of about 50 researchers and physicians gathered in a large auditorium and were tasked with evaluating the cost of reagents and equipment to undertake the AIDS studies. They decided to propose a $2.9 million budget, though Jay was haunted by the difficulty of getting any funding and said the proposal should be much less – as low as $1.2 million. But the others resisted and one bellowed, "Sit down Levy, we need this funding!" The proposal stayed at $2.9 million.

The following month, the bill passed and the funds were released. "I was amazed by the speed with which the money was approved," recalls Jay. "It was very encouraging to all of us who were prepared to work on this new epidemic."

But once again, Jay faced a barrier: the money approved for UCSF – $190,000 – was seized by Schmid, the UCSF dean. (This did not happen at any of the other schools that received funds.) He wouldn't release the money, saying a committee of experts needed to approve it. It was a surprising decision given that Jay had just published a paper about AIDS in *The Lancet*, a highly respected medical journal, and most of the researchers on the UCSF proposal had other NIH-approved grants.

Schmid gave a technocratic justification for why the state-allocated funds couldn't go straight to UCSF even though the legislature had directed that the funds bypass each school's leadership. The delay attracted notice and was even the subject of a *San Francisco Chronicle* article.31[31] Jay later wrote, "It became obvious to us that the administration really did not want to support our efforts." And this lack of support, said Jay, "certainly hindered my early work as well as that of others."[32]

A few weeks later, Schmid came to Jay's office with a map of the space on the 12th floor and said a room being used by Jay needed to be reassigned, for another project. When Jay defended the need for all his space, Schmid threatened to seize the room and pre-emptively sent him a memo thanking him for relinquishing the space. The notice was sent to a long list of other UCSF faculty. Jay refused, explained why in a note to Schmid, and copied all of the recipients of Schmid's original memo. Schmid nonetheless said he would have the equipment removed.

On the day this was scheduled to happen, Jay plastered a large sign with a biosafety label on the door to this lab that read, "HIV Research – Biosafety notice – Do Not Enter." The tactic worked – nothing was removed. Soon thereafter, Jay gave a well-received talk to the Department of Medicine about his AIDS research. Schmid liked the talk and eventually gave Jay an additional lab to undertake his studies.

UCSF's obstinacy was one of many institutions that manufactured reasons not to support AIDS research. Randy Shilts, a San Francisco journalist and the author of an authoritative book about the early years of AIDS, wrote that,

> In those early years, the federal government viewed AIDS as a budget problem, local public health officials saw it as a political problem, gay leaders considered AIDS a public relations problem, and the news media regarded it as a homosexual problem that wouldn't interest anybody else. Consequently, few confronted AIDS for what it was, a profoundly threatening medical crisis.[33]

The episode was emblematic of UCSF's posture at the time. As Jay has said of the school's administration,

> They were afraid we would not get the best medical students, the best interns, and [the best] residents so the aim was to keep our

> efforts a secret. As a result, the few of us who were initially involved in GRID formed a tight unit working together. In this regard, there was a moment, early in our studies, that the Dean at that time called me to the office to tell me that he did not want to see any publicity on AIDS. This he said was not necessary and was not what UCSF should become known for. UCSF's head of public relations was not pleased. And so while UCSF continued to make important contributions to information on AIDS, the publicity about these contributions was limited.

The resistance Jay encountered from UCSF's leadership on the AIDS epidemic, which was hitting San Francisco especially hard, could have been a catalyst for him to take his knowledge to another institution. But doing so would have delayed his research at precisely the moment when he was unlocking new insights about HIV and AIDS. His perseverance, after much controversy, would soon be recognized – for him professionally and for public understanding of the deadly condition.

Chapter 8

The Quest to Pinpoint the Cause of AIDS

In Jay's 1981 talk at San Francisco General, he explained why, if KS was caused by a cytomegalovirus (a leading idea for a virus causing this cancer), the virus would not be removed. As he later recounted,

> I went back to the fact that if a DNA virus was causing the cancer, it would be locked in the cell and wouldn't express the total particle. Similar to lysogeny and bacteriophages, the virus replicates in the cell, and kills the cell. This disease did not feature a strong cell death. I said it might be a defective cytomegalovirus and that we would like to work on this problem. But I had no money.

Jay also said a herpes virus could be the cause of KS. During his time in Uganda, while in medical school, he had seen electron microscopic (EM) pictures of Kaposi's sarcoma tissues in which a herpes virus could be recognized. At the time, he and others believed this was the human herpes simplex virus replicating in a growing tumor.

Jay was particularly interested in finding viruses that could convert cells into cancer cells, which made Volberding's phone call timely. In fact, Jay had worked with RNA tumor viruses at NIH that were associated with cancers and immune deficiency in animals. Notably, it was not yet known that a new herpesvirus (HHV 8) was the cause of KS.[34]

In the early 1980s, one of the fundamental challenges for all researchers was trying to pinpoint the agent that caused AIDS. Every Thursday morning, Jay would meet with others who shared his interest in discovering the causative agent. The meetings included infectious disease clinicians, scientists, epidemiologists, biostatisticians, students, and postdocs – all interested in determining why KS was now a major illness particularly in the young population that had never been seen before.

Jay believed the cause of the immune deficiency was a new human virus. Larry Drew and others thought it might be a mutant of CMV or even hepatitis B. Others had ideas on toxins or behavior. "The discussions were lively, informative and helpful," recalls Jay, "bringing many diverse groups together to try to determine the cause of AIDS."

One theory was that the agent came from Haiti, since the Haitian population in Florida had a high prevalence of AIDS. In December 1982, Jay visited Haiti (his sister lived in the Dominican Republic, which is on the same island as Haiti). It was thought that animals could be a carrier of the virus, but there were few wild animals in Haiti (nearly all of them had been killed for food). Jay has recounted the details of his visit:

> We decided to see if there was something in a voodoo ceremony that might lead to passage of an infectious agent. Although only chickens were involved we paid a voodoo priest to hold a ceremony in December. Not surprisingly, there was nothing that suggested a way for the emergence of an infectious agent causing AIDS. Nevertheless, when I was in Haiti I was told that Port-au-Prince was a frequent holiday destination for the gay population in New York. Therefore, the virus could have come from NY. This could have been in 1978, four years prior to my visit to the country. Much later when we brought back HIV isolates from Haiti and compared them to viruses circulating in the United States, they were very

> similar in genetic sequence both viral groups were Clade B. Of course, the virus could have come from Africa via Haiti and then to the States through New York. That possibility of transmission as early as 1978 has not been fully evaluated.[35]

A few months after that visit to Haiti, Jay was invited to a town meeting in San Francisco to discuss HIV. During the meeting, he noted that in Africa the virus could be spread by witch doctors who used unsterilized instruments for scarification. During the question-and-answer period, a young girl who had been raised in Africa stood up and chastised Jay for referencing a "witch doctor." She said, "In our country they are traditional doctors and we have faith in them."

"I was so embarrassed," recalls Jay, "particularly because I had worked in Africa in the 1960s and understood the importance of the traditional doctor. I apologized and hoped the crowd of 300 did not hold it against me – I was after all a young investigator just new at these public meetings."

In July 1983, Jay co-authored a paper in *The Lancet* that identified AIDS as an opportunistic infection that took advantage of a compromised immune system, though a reduced and enhanced immune response could be involved.[36] He later recounted,

> I originally thought that in individuals whose immune system was somewhat altered--i.e., babies, gay men who have used drugs, IV-drug people--the AIDS agent in most cases would be fought off, but there would be a group of people that would succumb. My thought was that the immune deficiency created an imbalance in the immune system, causing some elements of the immune system to overreact and produce cytokines that worked on

> increasing growth and transformation of endothelial cells, which are the origin of Kaposi's sarcoma. So I called AIDS a disease of hypo- and hyper-immune responses. I still believe that. It's just that the hyper-response which keeps emerging as an idea – autoimmune-type – isn't as prominent a problem as we might have expected. But Kaposi's sarcoma could be a result of a hyperactive immune system trying to respond to a deficit that has occurred because other elements of the immune system are decreased. And because we now know that herpesvirus 8 is responsible for KS, approaches at modifying the immune response have not yet been described.

Soon after Jay's paper was published in *The Lancet*, the UCSF administration released the $190,000 in state funding to him. He bought the ultracentrifuge the following month, which enabled him to begin concentrating possible virus particles in culture fluids and doing reverse transcriptase and other assays for detecting a virus. These procedures were fundamental to Jay's research.

> When we first did those studies, we used 7 milliliters of blood from a Wesleyan friend who had been a year ahead of me in college and who had just been diagnosed with AIDS. He came to my lab with a tube of his blood and wished me luck in finding a virus. When we separated out his white blood cells, and put them in culture, their image had visually changed. It looked like they were dying or changing shape. In some cases, there were huge cells containing many nuclei – characteristic of cells formed by fusion of cell membranes. And because we finally had the ultracentrifuge, we

> could pellet these cells and conduct studies to determine whether a retrovirus was involved. Much to our amazement, the amount of the retroviral reverse transcript enzyme associated with this infection was very, very high, indicating that many viruses were being produced.

About four weeks after beginning to use the centrifuge, Jay, with the help of his virology colleagues in the Bay Area, was able to identify a retrovirus by electron microscopy. The eccentric nucleus of the virus further indicated it was a member of the lentivirus subfamily. This was a significant breakthrough in the understanding of HIV, but rather than publicize it, Schmid, the school's Dean, held firm: "We are not going to be an AIDS University," he told Jay.

As noted above, when Jay arrived at UCSF he had organized a group of virologists in the Bay Area from UC-Berkeley, the Stanford VA Hospital, and other UC faculty, to form a group called the Tumor and Virus Group of the West. (Its euphemistic abbreviation, which was suggested by UC-Berkeley's Walter Nelson-Rees, was TuViGrouWe.) Besides EM pictures, they performed studies that indicated that the major target of the virus was a CD4 lymphocyte. Subsequent immunofluorescence antibody studies using HIV-infected cells confirmed that the patient had antibodies to the AIDS virus in his blood. This assay resembled that which Jay used to study antibodies to EBV in Burkitt lymphoma patients in Africa. Larry Kaminsky, a resident from the dermatology department, could undertake this test in as little as 20 minutes.

The results indicated a retrovirus, "but I wasn't expecting *that* virus," recalls Jay. "I asked myself if it was possible that a retrovirus could survive the purification of clotting factors VIII and IX in blood? Could they survive the commercial production of these factors for therapy? Was this a virus that could cause AIDS in hemophiliacs? This could be a different type of virus." As noted above, when Jay and his team sent the white cells for electron microscopy, they saw a virus that had the shape of a retrovirus, but it had an eccentric nucleus, which was a characteristic of a lentivirus.

Jay's research team then injected the AIDS-associated Retrovirus 2 (ARV-2) into small animals, to see if this was an agent that would cause immune destruction. The animals were housed seven miles away in a location that was highly protected for possibly dangerous microbes. After several weeks of observation, none of these animals showed any sign of a viral infection. Later, one of Jay's former virology colleagues from Texas, Sy Kalter, told Jay he could provide a chimpanzee from the Southwest Research Institute for the AIDS virus injection. After a few months, they found that the chimpanzee had been infected by this lentivirus by showing antibodies in the immunofluorescence assay established in the Levy lab. These results indicated that the ARV-2 had definitely infected the chimpanzee that then had a reaction against the virus. But over the next few years, there was never any clinical evidence of a viral infection.

Chapter 9

Research Breakthroughs and a Tussle with NIH

HIV creates an environment in which immune deficiency can occur (remember that AIDS stands for "Acquired Immune Deficiency Syndrome"). And in this immuno-compromised state, opportunistic infections and cancers can develop.

But that wasn't fully understood at the time. And Jay's paper on AIDS as an opportunistic infection was published shortly after a group of virologists at the Pasteur Institute, headed by Luc Montagnier, published a breakthrough paper in *Science*. They suggested a retrovirus, which they called "LAV," for lymphadenopathy-associated virus, was the cause of AIDS.[37] They considered it related to the human T-cell leukemia virus (HTLV), which had been isolated by a group at the National Institutes of Health led by Robert Gallo. (By coincidence, Jay had worked at the Pasteur Institute in Paris with the French researchers in 1978-80 and he wrote to them and congratulated them on finding this virus.) Soon after, the Gallo-led NIH group reported finding HTLV in AIDS patients and the assumption was that HTLV was very similar to the LAV virus found by the French.

But Jay was skeptical that this virus was the cause of AIDS since it was associated with T-cell leukemia. And that meant HTLV could not cause AIDS because that virus *transformed* white blood cells into cancer cells whereas the AIDS virus *killed* cells, particularly CD4+ lymphocytes. "When I discussed this in a commentary," recalls Jay, "it irritated Gallo, who was convinced that this new disease was caused by HTLV." This was the first of several instances in which Gallo tried to claim credit for finding the cause of AIDS.

That was the backdrop to a breakthrough Jay achieved in November 1983. He isolated a different retrovirus from several AIDS patients, including gay men, who did not show the disease. As noted above, he called this virus the AIDS-associated Retrovirus (ARV). This finding, which was enabled by cell culture and biochemical approaches Jay had used in studying other viruses, was the first isolation of this type of virus from an American patient. "It expanded the focus on characterization of this human retrovirus, while also giving rise to new approaches to detect and combat it through treatment and prevention," recalls Jay.

The breakthrough had been delayed by a year because Jay did not have access to the centrifuge, nor the filter on the hood. He also wanted to be certain that the agent he found associated with AIDS was linked to this disease in all the risk groups including hemophiliacs. Thus, he waited for the results on the clotting factor experiments before announcing his discovery. Those results involved adding a retrovirus to clotting factor concentrates when the treatment with results became available, in March 1984. ARV was resistant to the treatment procedures. Then Jay realized that a retrovirus was strongly associated with AIDS in hemophiliacs. He did not relate the virus findings to the French or NIH isolates because the reagents identifying each of these viruses had not yet been available.

Jay's results on ARV were published in *Science* in August 1984.[38] What should have been a landmark publication was overshadowed by Gallo. Three months earlier, he had four papers on his retrovirus published in *Science* simultaneously. Instead of recognizing the agent as a new retrovirus, Gallo and his NIH colleagues again concluded, mistakenly, that it was related to HTLV.

Jay wanted to determine if an ARV was related to either of the other AIDS viruses (e.g. LAV, HTLV -3), which depended on the specific reagents or identification of what made them unique. Gallo, as noted above, received Jay's letter asking for the antiserum to HTLV-3 but was angry with him. "It now seems obvious," says Jay, "that if he had sent his antisera, the ARV's would have been shown to be completely different retroviruses."

Gallo greatly benefited from being at NIH, which is an arm of the US government. The Reagan Administration, which gave little attention to AIDS as well as the causative agent, wanted to take credit for the achievement. Gallo's announcement led Margaret Heckler, the Secretary of the Department of Health and Human Services (which oversees NIH), to hold a press conference two weeks before his papers were published. She declared that "the probable cause of AIDS has been found, a variant of a known human cancer retrovirus called HTLV-3." She credited Gallo for the "breakthrough" and had him speak at the press conference.

But there was no mention of research conducted by Montagnier and others at the Pasteur Institute that had already been published. Three of the papers focused on the isolation and partial characterization of the retrovirus. The fourth paper focused on a way to test for the presence of antibodies to HTLV-3 in human blood. (The Department of Health and Human Services had applied for a patent on this test a month earlier.)

Those results attracted considerable media coverage, though Montagnier and others at the Pasteur Institute later claimed that Gallo's results were less impressive than they seemed. The Pasteur Institute researchers sent Gallo their LAV and they asserted that he did nothing more than reisolate the same virus that they had linked to AIDS. More than a decade later, *Science* acknowledged that "subsequent sequencing of the genomes of Gallo's and Montagnier's viruses showed they were sufficiently similar to be identical."[39] That observation had also been made by the studies of Marty Bryant in Murray Gardener's lab.[40]

In contrast to Gallo, who had worked with the French virus (which he claims he did not receive), Jay never had access to it. That made his achievement even more noteworthy. He had limited funds and a small staff and grew the isolated virus in cell culture himself. Notably, when the Gallo's papers were published, Jay immediately wrote to him and requested his reagents, saying that his studies of AIDS in San Francisco revealed that, "we have also isolated retroviruses and now would like to know if any of them are related to HTLV-3." Gallo never responded.

Jay was once again undermined by his university's reluctance to publicize his findings. Just a few days after Gallo's papers were published in *Science*, Jay gave a lecture at a joint meeting of the American Society for Clinical Oncology and the American Association for Cancer Research on viruses and autoimmunity and immune disorders. He shared his ARV data on the AIDS-associated retrovirus, ARV. One speaker approached him after and said, "Jay, I can't get over all the data you have. Why haven't you spoken about it?"[41]

Though it was written up in a Canadian newspaper, as well as the *San Francisco Examiner* and the *San Francisco Chronicle*, Jay was worried that if the data attracted too much attention his paper wouldn't be accepted for publication in *Science* (medical journals want breakthrough findings to appear there first). He also asked UCSF about holding a press conference to publicize his findings. He was told they didn't want any media coverage about this work. "The Dean didn't like any publicity on AIDS," Jay later recalled. "The school was afraid to have any attention given to this disease for fear it would compromise chances of getting good house staff. Many young people might avoid a medical school closely associated with AIDS."

Jay knew that it was important to keep Gallo informed of his work, since he had influence with senior leaders in the science community. He always found Gallo cordial and welcome. But he also knew him as a polarizing and highly controversial figure in science. Jay recalls that Gallo went to great lengths to diminish the significance of his findings, sought to block the publication of one of his papers, and tried to prevent him from speaking at an international conference on HIV/AIDS.

Soon after Jay's paper was published in *Science*, he was invited to give a lecture at NIH organized by the HIV/retrovirus group there and discuss his findings on the possible AIDS virus. While at NIH, he met with a former colleague, Malcolm Martin, who asked to hear about his work. After Jay described his group's isolation of the AIDS virus and the antibody studies, Martin replied, "Jay, you need to be careful. I just came from a meeting at UC Davis and Murray Gardner's group presented evidence that indicated that LAV from Montagnier and HTLV-III from Gallo are very similar but your virus is totally different. That places your virus outside the general common characteristics of the other isolates. Could it be a maverick?"

When Jay told him that his group had several isolates that were examined by Southern blot and that they were all different, Martin said, "Oh my God." He recognized that LAV and HTLV-III were the same virus. In other words, Gallo re-isolated the virus that Montagnier had sent him. Jay later wrote,

> This fact was soon supported by several other observations such as the electron microscopic picture of HTLV-III published by Gallo that had been labeled on the photo in his lab, LAV. . . . While the Gallo group said they had not received LAV at any time, Montag-

> nier claimed he had sent it at least five times. Now the proof was there. For some reason, I think politically, that information was never widely appreciated, stated or greatly considered. Some have said that it was hushed up by the NIH. Instead, Gallo and Montagnier, for some reason, signed an agreement stating that they found the virus at about the same time. The work of our group, without any receipt of a sample virus from the French, independently discovered the AIDS-associated retroviruses (ARV).
>
> However, our observations and our publication (just 3 months after the Gallo papers) were not well-cited. . . .. Our work continued and there were many examples told to me by individuals that NIH would take my name off invitations to conferences and one journal editor was threatened to not receive any submissions from the Gallo lab if it accepted my review on retroviruses. Fortunately, the paper was accepted and published anyway.[42]

Therefore, it was scientifically proven that the French virus, LAV, was the first virus found to have an association with AIDS; the UCSF isolate from the Levy lab was the first virus isolated from an American patient. These two retroviruses were genetically distinct.

What ensued was a battle for recognition of each investigator's role in scientific discovery. As is often seen in the history of science, things got personal.

Jay remembers that in 1985, Gallo called him saying he would refuse to cite any of Jay's work unless he would agree to identify Gallo as a co-discoverer of HIV. "During the call, he also tried to convince me to accept the name of the AIDS virus as HTLV 3/ARV or ARV/HTLV-3," recalls Jay. "I said that there was no way I could accept that suggestion since it was clear that the French had discovered the virus first and their name should be considered." Gallo replied by asking, "Jay, where is your national loyalty?"

During the call, Jay explained that his team had its isolates by November 1983. Gallo countered by saying he found his virus in 1982, though there's strong evidence he was working with the French virus, not a unique virus. "I noted that we felt we definitely confirmed the isolation of a retrovirus that resembled that found by the French," recalls Jay. "Whether it was the same one or different one needed further study." Gallo asked why Jay had not attempted to determine if the viruses Jay had found were similar to HTLV-3. "I reminded him that I had written to him and requesting anti-sera to his virus but he did not respond," recalls Jay. "He admitted that he received my letter but was angry with me and so he did not send the serum."

One month later, in April 1985, Jay attended the first International AIDS Conference, which was held in Atlanta. He was not invited to give a major plenary lecture (while Gallo was) and his work was barely mentioned. "I was disappointed not to be given credit for finding the AIDS virus," he recalls. The conference proceedings focused on the French discovery versus the NIH observations. At a reception during the conference, an NIH researcher named Mikulas Popovic challenged Jay for not accepting the findings of the Gallo lab. Popovic then cussed at Jay and punched him repeatedly, while yelling epithets. There were no repercussions for Popovic.

Jay had less contact with Gallo in the years that followed, but as leading virologists they remained visible to each other. In 1995, Gallo reviewed Jay's book, *HIV and the Pathogenesis of AIDS,* in a medical journal, *Trends in Microbiology.*[43] He described Jay as "one of the chief contributors to our understanding of the pathogenesis of HIV-induced disease" and said the book "will be valuable to a wide range of students of this disease." He also praised several elements of the book, such as the exploration of HIV transmission and the effects of HIV on individual organs.

But most of the review was devoted to criticizing the book. Some of it was nit-picking, such as quibbling with some of Jay's citations. But the more sweeping critique – what Gallo characterized as a "serious flaw" – covered Jay's history of the HIV discovery. Gallo was irked that his research was not cited, saying that, "the treatment here is not close to the accurate and careful treatment of other subjects" in the book.

The jab was a reminder (if any was needed) of Gallo's campaign to put himself at the center of HIV-AIDS history.

Chapter 10

A Life-Saving Discovery

Hemophiliacs were among the most vulnerable groups in the early days of AIDS. They are born without the proteins known as Factor VIII and IX, which are essential for blood to clot. In the 1970s, medications known as "factor concentrate" enabled blood clotting and they could be taken at home as a preventive measure. Factor concentrate was created by obtaining human blood plasma from up to 40,000 people and extracting the required clotting factor.

The development of factor concentrates also enabled hemophiliacs to get surgeries and other procedures that would have been unthinkable in the past. As one physician working on hemophilia observed, "It seemed that hemophilia treatment had never been better." But the good times wouldn't last, he wrote: "All of this changed when AIDS made its way into the blood supply."[44]

There was always a risk that even a tiny amount of contamination in the plasma could sharply increase the risk of a virus infection. And inadequate testing for HIV led to hemophiliacs using contaminated factor concentrate products. Nearly 5,000 hemophiliacs were infected with HIV before concentrates were deemed safe and more than 4,000 of them eventually died of AIDS.

One of Jay's most important discoveries was demonstrating how to use heat to inactivate HIV in clotting factor preparations. His research involved clotting factor treatments for hemophilia, Factor VIII and Factor IX. This procedure did not affect the clotting factor levels. Thus the approach could be used to obtain virus-free clotting factors.

The results surprised Jay. "I had worked with mouse retroviruses and I knew they were very sensitive to physical and biochemical treatments. If you lyophilized them, freeze-dried them, you could keep them active, but they lost some infectivity," he later said. "I felt that the procedures for preparing Factor VIII would probably inactivate the virus. How then could a retrovirus cause AIDS since the chance of this virus surviving Factor VIII preparation would be low?"

He called an acquaintance at the Centers for Disease Control, Bruce Evatt, and asked whether all hemophiliacs with AIDS had received whole blood transfusions. If they had, surmised Jay, then his idea would go nowhere, because they could get the virus from blood transfusions. But it turned out that some hemophiliacs only got Factor VIII concentrate and they too had AIDS. The cause, therefore, had to be in the factor treatment.

In the fall of 1983, Jay set out to test this idea. As he later explained,

> I wanted to determine what this virus was, and how to eliminate it. The RT assay suggested a retrovirus and I felt passing the virus-containing fluid through factor purification procedures would inactivate the virus. This could be expected since it would be subjected to acid, pH changes, filtration, pelleting, centrifugation. All of these procedures should inactivate the virus but leave viable factor products for hemophiliacs.

He contacted five companies manufacturing Factor VIII. He wanted to have them prepare the clotting factor in fluids with mouse retroviruses according to their procedures and see what happened to it. He also wanted to determine if there was a different virus that would not survive Factor

VIII treatments. Four of the companies said they couldn't work with him, because their procedure was under patent (even though he wasn't asking them to reveal any secrets). More generally, they simply didn't want to be involved with the research with this "dangerous" virus. But one company, Cutter, which was a subdivision of Miles Laboratory and based nearby in Emeryville, agreed to collaborate with Jay.

Starting in late 1983, Jay conducted experiments with mouse retroviruses. He would send the mouse viruses to Cutter lab to place into Factor VIII containing fluid. The company would then bring it back to UCSF, and Jay's lab would measure how much of the virus remained after the Factor VIII was purified. They also checked the sensitivity of the virus to heat treatment. They found that it took up to 72 hours at 68 degrees C. to kill all the mouse viruses remaining in the lyophilized product. The study, which was completed in March 1984, showed that the mouse retrovirus could survive in the freeze-dried product. Importantly, the clotting factors were resistant to heat treatment.

This important discovery, which was later the basis of a paper published in *The Lancet*,[45] prompted Jay and the Cutter research team to contact the National Hemophilia Foundation. They recommended that the foundation immediately adopt heat treatment as the accepted therapy with clotting factors for hemophilia. But the foundation refused, saying that the research was only done with a mouse virus, not a human virus. Jay thought that another reason the foundation didn't accept the recommendation was that it would have had to endorse a recall of all the clotting factor products and have them heat-treated. That would have cost millions of dollars.

The findings from Jay and Cutter were published in the CDC's Morbidity and Mortality Weekly Report in October 1984.[46] Evatt, the CDC official who was involved with heat treatment, later authored a paper in which he recounted what happened after the CDC released its findings.

> The world's hemophilia community quickly adopted the [Medical and Scientific Advisory Council of the National Hemophilia Foundation] recommendation, so that by the beginning of 1985 little non-heated clotting FVIII was used anywhere. The AIDS epidemic in the hemophilic patients thus suddenly ceased. Subsequent studies of birth cohorts demonstrated that no hemophilic patients, born in the USA in 1985 and later, were infected with LAV, later to be renamed HIV. Tragically, during the period 1981 to 1984, more than 50 percent of the population of hemophilic patients in the USA had already become infected and these individuals would continue to present clinical symptoms of AIDS during the next decade and many would die.[47]

Jay recognized that before all hemophiliacs would be protected, he needed to determine similar inactivation of a human retrovirus could be demonstrated. To do so, his research team took blood from a healthy person and spiked it with high amounts of a human retrovirus (ARV 2). Predictably, they found this virus was also very sensitive to heat treatment. This was 6-9 months after Jay's team had made the same observation with the mouse virus.

One of Jay's great regrets, he now says, is that "I should have been more forceful in stating to the clotting factor companies that they should heat all their products immediately by the procedures we had used in the lab studies. Had they done this, it could have prevented many thousand hemophiliacs from becoming infected."

Almost immediately, hospitals and other medical centers used three days of heat treatment to eliminate the virus. But scientific journals were reluctant to publish the result, saying Jay and his team were just repeating the mouse work. The reviewers did not appreciate the clinical importance of showing the human virus was also sensitive to heat. The result finally appeared in *The Lancet*, in June 1985, as a letter.[48] The CDC also conducted a study and reached a similar conclusion, which was published in December 1985.[49]

Jay's findings provided early evidence linking the potential for blood-borne transmission of retroviruses, like HIV, with the use of Factor VIII concentrates. This research contributed to the understanding of how retroviruses could be transmitted through blood products. It also led to the development of stricter screening and heat-treatment protocols for Factor VIII concentrates, which would prevent HIV transmission to hemophiliac patients. In 1986, Jay shared an award from the National Hemophilia Foundation for finding a way to make blood products safe.

Other discoveries

After Jay discovered the virus, he needed to evaluate its genetic structure. But at UCSF, he did not have access to the equipment he needed. When he approached a UCSF colleague, Bill Rutter, and told him about the dilemma, Rutter said the biotechnology company he had recently co-founded, Chiron, could provide what Jay needed. "I was uneasy," recalls Jay.

> I had been told throughout my career not to get involved with industry. In particular, I thought about how Wally Rowe, my mentor at NIH, would be disappointed in my decision to work with a commercial company. However, Bill said to me, 'with my

> company we could perform studies in a few months.' In our lab at UCSF, it could have taken two years. The decision was therefore quite easy, given that AIDS was now affecting many individuals in our city and state.

Fortunately, the company was located nearby, in Emeryville. "Its facilities were spectacular," says Jay. "I'd never seen equipment that modern." The equipment enabled Jay to fully evaluate the retrovirus. Working with people at Chiron such as Paul Luciw and Dino Dina, Jay was able to clone the virus – his group was the first to do so. Cloning made it possible to identify where HIV fits into the family of viruses.

Jay was also among the first to sequence an ARV isolate, which made it possible to know the structure of the virus as well as targets that would be used in developing a therapy. Sequencing also showed that all HIV isolates have a different sequence, making it possible to pinpoint if the virus had come from the same person or the same location.

Jay's sequencing demonstrated the diversity of AIDS viruses, and that the retrovirus isolated by Gallo at the NIH (HTLV-3) was the same as that isolated by Montagnier in Paris (LAV). Therefore, Jay's results indicated that the ARV isolates were the first AIDS human retroviruses identified in the United States and each had a different genetic makeup. None of them were similar to LAV.

Jay made one other critical discovery: some people infected with the virus remained healthy. He found that HIV replication was suppressed by immune CD8+ cells that produced an anti-HIV protein he called CAF (CD8+ Cell Antiviral Factor). Jay's lab has been focused on defining the nature of CAF for several years. This discovery about CD8+ cells and CAF gave encouragement to the world that a natural mechanism for control of the AIDS virus was now found. He identified these virus-suppressing cells of the immune system through an experiment involving the removal of CD8+ cells from an AIDS blood sample that had no evidence of HIV. Within a week, that culture he was using showed the presence of the virus. Those immune cells had antiviral activity. When they were added back to the culture, the virus disappeared.

"When we separated the CD8 cells from the effects of CD4 cells, we found HIV was suppressed by the culture fluid," recalls Jay. When we discovered this effect of CD8+ cells, I was as excited as I've ever been in HIV research."[50] But, he adds, "it has been difficult to determine the full nature of this antiviral activity."

Chapter 11

A Scientist Dissents and the Elusive Quest for a Vaccine

A perplexing episode unfolded while Jay was researching HIV-AIDS and it involved a good friend and a fellow scientist, Peter Duesberg.

Duesberg was a distinguished – and well respected – biochemist at UC-Berkeley, with a focus on the nexus between genes and cancer. He was a tenured professor and a member of the National Academy of Sciences. (He passed away in January 2026.)

Starting in 1987, Duesberg began publishing articles claiming that HIV did not cause AIDS and was harmless. AIDS, he argued, was triggered by taking recreational drugs or antiretroviral drugs. He did more than just publish academic papers. He peddled his message in the media, in mass market books, and in speeches at schools.

Jay felt somewhat responsible for Duesberg's belief that HIV did not cause AIDS. In a casual conversation, Jay mentioned that he had some patients who were infected with HIV but the virus couldn't be found. At that time, Jay had not yet discovered the non-cytotoxic antiviral response of CD8 cells in which the secretion of a CD8 antiviral factor (CAF) blocked virus release from the infected cells. "Part of Peter's reasoning was that not everyone showing HIV got sick and also that I could not isolate HIV from everyone who had AIDS," recalls Jay. "But he was leaving out the detail that removal of the CD8 cells will lead to release of the virus."

Duesberg had a book published in 1996, *Inventing the AIDS Virus*. It was reviewed in *The New York Times* by June Osborn, a microbiologist and the former chair of the National Commission on AIDS. "At the core of

Mr. Duesberg's thesis," wrote Osborn, "is his belief that, by definition, there can be no such thing as an illness induced by a virus that has its overt onset years after initial infection. Further, he asserts that no virus can cause more than a single disease, or any disease that appears after a neutralizing immune response develops." Osborn threw cold water on Duesberg's thesis: "This remarkable belief flies in the face of decades of progress in understanding infectious diseases."[51]

A comprehensive review of Duesberg's work, published in *Science*, led to a similar conclusion: "Mainstream AIDS researchers argue that Duesberg's arguments are constructed by a selective reading of the scientific literature, dismissing evidence that contradicts his theses, requiring impossibly definitive proof, and dismissing outright studies marked by inconsequential weaknesses."[52]

Jay recalls that, "people wanted me to challenge him, but I didn't want to. Peter was very good at manipulating words." Instead, Jay had Duesberg over to his house for a one-on-one meeting in the early 1990s and they talked for two hours. Jay presented all of the evidence showing the link between HIV and AIDS. At the conclusion of their meeting, Jay's wife, Sharon, came into the room to say hello. Duesberg said, "Sharon, I want you to know that Jay has convinced me more than ever that HIV is not the cause of AIDS."

Duesberg also called David Perlman of the *San Francisco Chronicle* the next morning to say that he had a meeting with Jay and implied that Jay had come around to believe his concepts – a complete fabrication.

> I called Peter and told him that he had disgraced our friendship. I was quite disappointed and did not have any more contact with him. He tried several times to get together again – we had enjoyed

> going with our wives to a San Francisco Greek restaurant, Salonika. We also had lab get-togethers, which were a great opportunity for my research involving biologic systems to interact with his research that dealt more with molecular biologic systems.

Given Duesberg's credentials, his contrarian views attracted outsized attention – and even affected public policy and safety. Thabo Mbeki, while president of South Africa from 1999-2008, embraced the Duesberg view that antiretroviral drugs contributed to the onset of AIDS. He delayed the introduction of an antiretroviral drug program and terminated government support of clinics that were using such drugs to prevent mother-to-child transmission of AIDS.

These policies carried a high cost. A study estimated that from 2000-05, more than 330,000 people died prematurely from HIV/AIDS as a result of the government blocking access to life-saving treatments. Moreover, at least 35,000 babies were born with HIV infections that could have been prevented.

The elusive quest for an HIV vaccine

For all the progress that's been made against AIDS, such as a 54 percent decline in mortality from AIDS-related illnesses since 2010, it's still a devastating disease. It was responsible for approximately 630,000 deaths in 2024[53] and it accounts for about 1.5 percent of deaths in the world each year.[54]

For more than 30 years, Jay's research has focused on trying to find a protein that could be the building block of a vaccine that would prevent HIV infection. He started the research with a built-in advantage. As noted earlier, he was the first to discover that some people infected with HIV remain healthy. Specifically, he found that HIV was suppressed by immune CD8+ cells that produce CAF (CD8+Cell Antiviral Factor).

Among people with detectable HIV In the blood, between 5 and 8 percent have normal CD4+ cells and low plasma viral levels. They do not experience the symptoms associated with AIDS. Some people have lived with HIV for more than 30 years, don't need medications, and have healthy immune systems.

These individuals, says Jay, have immune systems that have figured out how to resist the virus and block its ability to cause diseases. CAF is the key immune protein preventing the HIV from replicating. Thus, expressing this protein or factor is fundamental to developing a vaccine against HIV. "But we haven't been able to figure out the full nature and structure of the factor," says Jay, "and it's only produced in limited amounts by the CD8+ lymphocytes."

> CAF is produced at such low levels (a 1:4 dilution of CD8+ cell culture fluid only gives 50 percent suppression of HIV replication in cell culture). Its identification has not yet been achieved.
> After many years, using antibodies to known human proteins, immunologic detection techniques, and purified cellular factors, no human proteins linked to CD8+ cells have yet been found with the characteristics of CAF.

Research has been painstakingly slow. "You could devote your entire career to this and end up with nothing," concedes Jay. With several million proteins produced in the body, identifying CAF is a real challenge. To help in this effort, a group of volunteers are "elite controllers." Their CD8+

cells can produce high amounts of this valuable protein.

The key, says Jay, is to develop an approach that enables increased production of CAF using immune cells from the elite controllers that can produce low abundance proteins. This can be achieved by culturing their CD8+lymphocytes with certain chemicals that help induce secretion of CAF. However, once the protein has been made, its instability in the laboratory poses another challenge.

Pharmaceutical companies have largely abandoned the search for this protein that can block HIV replication, because they haven't seen any meaningful progress over the past 30 years. "It's a challenge that requires new thinking," says Jay.

That new thinking may come from artificial intelligence (AI). That approach has the potential to help identify the best chemicals to increase CAF production and help with the differential analysis of thousands of potential proteins in cultures that look at anti-HIV activity. "I am confident that progress in cell culture and protein production will uncover the identity of CAF and enable its high production," says Jay. "It is very possible that a *beshert* moment will uncover this unexpected antiviral activity associated with a specific or previously unknown human protein."

Chapter 12

Vignettes

Scientific discovery has been central to Jay's adult life – but so have other forms of discovery. He has traveled widely throughout the world, had innumerable adventures along the way, and met many notable characters (both famous and unknown). Details from some of these (mostly non-scientific) discoveries are collected here.

Meeting Muhammad Ali

Jay spent the summer after his third year in medical school in Uganda. His flight on Pan Am allowed for a stopover in Cairo, where he visited a local medical school. He also traveled to see the pyramids. While he was climbing the Second Great Pyramid, he heard shouting and loud noises coming from the nearby Sphinx. A crowd had assembled and was following a young man in a flowing white robe. The man began to climb the Sphinx, which wasn't permitted, and when Jay was able to see the man's face, he recognized him: it was Muhammad Ali, the world famous boxer.

When Ali reached the platform of the Sphinx, Jay waved vigorously and cried out, "Cassius! Cassius!" Ali waved back and shouted, "It's Muhammad, Muhammad!" (Ali had changed his name from Cassius Clay.) Jay then raced down the pyramid and ran toward the Sphinx. "Amazingly, the crowd parted to make a path for me," recalls Jay, "probably believing that I was a friend of his."

Ali came down from the platform and greeted Jay. They chatted about what they were each doing in Cairo and then Jay handed his camera to a reporter who was following Ali and they got a picture together. As Ali walked away, through the large crowd, he shouted to Jay, "Send me the photos!" Jay tried, but never found an address.

Trying to buy an abandoned French village

In 1971, Jay was temporarily based in Paris while he waited for the renovation of his UCSF lab to be completed. He was working with Professor Michel Boiron at Hospital Saint-Louis in the 10th district. Jay was there to teach retrovirology to researchers and they were focused on studying mouse viruses that could infect human cells. Jay's friends included the professor's son, Olivier, and a friend of Olivier, Bertrand, as well as Bertrand's girlfriend, Nena. "We would go to cafes and meet young people," recalls Jay. "I enjoyed their *joie de vivre.*"

During one of their nights out, a member of their group shared the information that there were entire villages for sale in a picturesque area of southeastern France called Ardèche. The group decided they should explore the unorthodox opportunity of purchasing a town. Before long, they'd set out on the drive and accompanying Jay was his girlfriend at the time, Nathalie Halphen, while Olivier, Nena, and Bertran drove in a separate car.

The young students were particularly interested in a village for sale named Bolze (pronounced "Balls"). To get there, they needed to start in a small town of about 1,300 people named Joyeuse, which translates as "joyous." Jay had all kinds of ideas for how to commercialize the village, cheekily playing on the "joyous" and "balls" imagery.

When they reached Joyeuse, they checked into a small inn and spoke with the owner about their trip. She was surprised by their interest and told them that villages around Joyeuse were completely abandoned, consisting of nothing more than rocks. The group insisted on seeing the village site and speaking with someone who had lived in the town. She told them there was an elderly local widow who might have information about Bolze.

Jay and Nathalie drove to see the woman in her apartment. Upon knocking on her door, she called from within and asked who was there – "*Qui est?*" – and what they wanted. Jay responded, in French, "My relatives once lived in a small village nearby called Bolze and I wanted to go look at it." A voice from within the apartment inquired as to the name of his relatives. "Blanc," Jay answered – knowing that a name like Levy would not be in this town. Therefore, he chose his mother's maiden name, Blank.

The widow bellowed from within, *"Oh! Les Blancs de Bolze!"* Much to Jay's surprise, there had been a family named Blanc who had lived in the village – a classic *beshert* moment. The widow's home health aide opened the door and showed them into the apartment. After some friendly discussion, Jay pretended to be related to the Blanc family of Bolze and identified himself as a doctor in San Francisco. The woman then took out a map of the region and marked the spot where Bolze was located. There were several abandoned homes (no one was living in Bolze). The woman marked the pathway leading to the village and warned them that it was a difficult two-kilometer walk, as no road was left.

Jay and Nathalie immediately returned to the inn and told the owner the good news. They showed her a copy of the map and she directed them to the path that would lead to the village. After a lunch that included the well-known white asparagus from the region, the five of them hiked on to find Bolze.

The walk was not difficult but required climbing over rocks and around bushes. It was easy to identify the village since it was located on about five hectares of land and had several houses indicated by fallen stones. A brook ran through the center of town and a few yards away was a prominent house, which is likely where the mayor lived. "I looked it over and wondered about living there," recalls Jay. They had a picnic with cheese sandwiches and red wine. Jay had brought a canvas, on which he made a painting of the village. "It was an exciting adventure and everyone in our group enjoyed dreaming about resurrecting this village," recalls Jay.

Jay and the others returned in a few days to the widow's apartment to learn more. She referred them to one of the village's former residents, a gentleman whose family had been prominent residents of Bolze. The group visited him in a retirement home in Joyeuse. The interaction was cordial. When Jay and Nathalie asked for the price, he said, *"quinze mille francs"* (15,000 francs). Nathalie said they would be discussing this with the group and get back to him very soon.

After returning to Paris, they contacted their friends Olivier, Jean, and Thomas. They all agreed that it was quite a reasonable price at 15,000 francs (or about $2,700 per person), even though the village was only rocks.

But a few days later, the inn's manager called Jay at his lab in Paris and said that the man they'd met with, who was a part owner of the village, was upping the price of the village by a factor of five. "I said I was surprised and upset," recalls Jay. "After all, we were going to renovate an abandoned village."

The manager called again the following week and said, "well, M. Levy, in my opinion you, as a customer, presented to the man some questionable characteristics, such as coming from Paris, being a doctor and most importantly, having the wrong last name." (She knew Jay's last name was Levy, not Blanc.)

Jay was shocked, but the woman said the man felt they misunderstood his French. Jay reminded her that Nathalie was a witness to this conversation. "Bertrand and I were particularly disturbed by being tricked and immediately planned the return trip to Ardèche to present our case," recalls Jay. He, Nathalie, and Bertran did return a few weeks later and met with the man. "He was very stern and determined not to sell the property to us," recalls Jay.

The group returned to Paris in anger. But the outcome was not a big surprise for Jay. "I knew there was a lot of antisemitism in southern France. But I did not give that a thought when negotiating the price." And while not being able to buy the village was a huge disappointment, says Jay, "it made for a very entertaining adventure. The ups and downs of the episode were examples of *beshert* and emblematic of my time in France."

Twins travel

When Jay and Stuart were 58, their mother had a *beshert* moment in a beauty parlor in Wilmington, Delaware. A woman friend in the parlor said she had heard about a 14-day, all-expenses paid cruise through the Panama Canal to commemorate the inauguration of a twin ship of the Dawn Princess (called the "Dawn Sunrise"). It would start and end in Fort Lauderdale, Florida. Passengers were chosen from applications and the criteria for eligibility was that the applicants needed to be contributing to people's lives besides being identical twins.

Stuart applied on behalf of himself and Jay. Much to their delight, they were chosen – perhaps because they were both physicians doing humanitarian work and because they still looked almost identical (photos were part of the application). "We knew we should not refuse the amazing trip," recalls Jay, "but we wanted to keep it a secret from our colleagues, since the concept was a bit hokey." (Upon arriving in Fort Lauderdale, they both went to a barber to get similar haircuts and Stuart had his mustache shaved off.)

Others in attendance were the original "Toni twins," who had appeared in television commercials; the so-called "Doublemint twins," who had appeared in ads for Wrigley chewing gum; the Josephson twins, who in 1988 and 1992 had won Olympic medals in synchronized swimming; and the Borden twins, blonde-haired women who had appeared in numerous television shows, including "I Love Lucy."

To thank the cruise ship and the passengers for being so nice to the invitees, the twins put on a variety show a few nights before the end of their trip. Jay and Stuart played their ukuleles and sang songs of the Highwaymen, who were schoolmates of Jay from Wesleyan.

"The trip may have been the best seven days of my life," recalls Jay. "I made a lot of new friends." Six of the sets of twins later came to a 60th birthday party for Jay and Stuart in San Francisco. (Jay and Stuart did not want anyone from UCSF or Tufts to know that they were on the trip, so they were a bit alarmed when they appeared in color photos on the front page of a Florida newspaper.)

Weizmann Institute

In 1979, Jay had a sabbatical from UCSF, and he chose to spend the time in Israel at the Weizmann Institute – one of the world's leading multidisciplinary basic research institutions in the natural and exact sciences. "I was inspired by people at Weizmann such as Michael Sela and Nechama Haran-Ghera," recalls Jay. "They were both pioneering scientists and role models for me. And the institute had a reputation for fostering innovative basic science thinking."

Sela later developed a drug to treat MS and Haran-Ghera, with whom Jay studied while at the institute, was an expert on radiation-induced cancer, particularly in mice, and pre-leukemic cells. Together, they researched the involvement of retroviruses in malignant transformation. "That led me to become cognizant of technologies involved in cell transformation," recalls Jay. "I also deepened my knowledge of retroviruses and their role in irradiation-induced leukemias in mice and other cancers."

While at the institute, Jay met many senior scientists and junior laboratory workers, some of whom he would later collaborate with in his studies of viruses and cancer. They included Leo Sachs, Yaron Cohen, Michael Walker, and Esther Hayes.

While in Israel, Jay swam in the Mediterranean. Soon thereafter, he came down with the hepatitis A virus, which he attributed to the presence of sewage in the sea. He was out of the lab for about two months, but he says the experience at Weizmann was still "wonderful," with Haran-Ghera becoming both a mentor and a good friend who Jay considered part of his extended family.

Jay wanted to improve his Hebrew while in Israel and he was tutored by a student in the Haran-Ghera lab, Michael Zeira. Michael also took Jay and Sharon on trips throughout Israel. Several years later, Michael was diagnosed with a tumor in his pituitary gland. At the time, there were only a few people in the world who operated on such tumors – one of them, Charlie Wilson, was a colleague of Jay's at UCSF. Jay contacted Wilson to inquire about operating on Zeira. Wilson said he would do it. When Jay asked about the fees, given the number of staff who would have to be involved, Wilson simply said that he would be sure that the hospital would cover the cost.

The operation was a success, and Wilson told Jay after the operation that he could deliver the good news to Zeira and his wife, Evelyn. They had been unable to conceive prior to the surgery (a likely product of the pituitary issue). But following the surgery, Evelyn was able to have two children, a son and a daughter. "My being at UCSF with one of the few people who operated on tumors in the pituitary gland was a great *beshert* moment," says Jay. "It gave Michael a new life and enabled him and Evelyn to bring children into the world."

When Jay returned to California, he was invited by a committee of the Weizmann Institute to give a talk and describe his experiences there. Soon after, the head of the institute's American committee, Helen Diller, invited him for lunch and proposed he take over for her in heading up the committee in the Bay Area. He said yes and stayed in that role for 10 years.

In 2013, Jay was elected president of the institute's American committee. In this capacity, he attended national and international committee meetings and worked with others on committee activities. He retired from the presidency in 2020 and has remained active in the institute's research activities.

In yet another example of *beshert*, the relationship with Helen Diller led to a deep and close friendship with Diller's daughter, Jackie, and Jackie's husband, Dan Safier. Their support helped to make this book possible.

A lab visit, and a dinner, with Sharon Stone

One day in 1999, a staff member from the American Foundation for AIDS Research (known as "amfAR"), where Jay served on the scientific advisory board for a decade, called Jay to say that Sharon Stone, the actress, would be coming to visit his AIDS lab. Jay and his colleagues were told not to expect her to stay very long and that photos should not be taken. She arrived with an assistant and was given what became known as the "Sharon Stone tour," which involved dressing in a protective gown, using a mask and gloves, and looking at HIV-infected cells through a microscope. She understood visualizing the destruction of cells and how they fused together to form a large cell containing many cell nuclei. She spoke with a long-term survivor who informed her of the activities of the gay community and how he felt as someone infected but showing no symptoms.

While exploring Jay's lab during the three-hour visit, someone asked if he could take a photo of her. She immediately said yes and then several photos were taken of her with Jay and his colleagues. She signed the bio-hood in Jay's lab.

About four hours after she departed, she called Jay. "She said that she had enjoyed the visit very much and was impressed by the dedication of my group," recalls Jay. "She wanted to give a dinner party in our honor and hoped that we would accept. I was really thrilled and of course accepted."

That event was at her home on 25th Avenue, where she lived with her husband at the time, Phil Bronstein, who was managing editor of the *San Francisco Examiner*. Jay drove his antique 1931 Citroen to the event. Stone marveled at its condition and Jay took her for a ride in it. Stone later became a strong advocate for HIV education and care and "an outstanding ambassador for the cause," recalls Jay.

A beshert *experience in Japan*

In the summer of 1964, Stuart had a fellowship to work in Japan with a Japanese scientist who worked in the field of resistance to drugs and antibiotics. When Stuart was on the plane going to Tokyo, a young redheaded student with a beard approached him and asked if he was Jay Levy. (This person had overlapped with Jay at Wesleyan.) Stuart and Jay were used to being confused and often played the opposite twin to avoid embarrassing the other person.

This time they ended up talking about why Stuart was going to Japan. The young man said he knew someone – Bu Yamashita – in Tokyo whom Stuart should meet. Stuart called Bu and went to his house. When his parents realized Stuart needed a place to stay, they invited him to stay with them for the duration of his two-month fellowship. It turns out Bu attended Williams and had met Stuart there. Bu's family owned the Yamashita shipping company, so Stuart had a very nice place to stay. "This was a classic *beshert* experience," observes Jay.

In 1965, Stuart asked Jay if he could show a young Japanese friend, Noburu, around New York. (Stuart had known Noburu from his time in Tokyo during the Olympics in Japan in 1964.) Noburu spent a day with Jay and his friends in New York and then returned to Japan. Jay later went to Japan to give a lecture at the Japan Cancer Society and Noburu took him on a tour of different places near Tokyo.

Noburu and his family would go on to play a large role in Jay's life. "I found the Japanese to be very well educated and very knowledgeable of events outside Japan," recalls Jay. Noburu's close friend, Taka (a nurse), and her husband, Iri (a rheumatologist), also became close friends of Jay and Stuart.

Noburu was immensely generous and starting in 1983 Jay and Sharon would take a trip with him to Japan every 10 years. In October 2023, they took a trip to Kyushu, the third-largest Japanese island. It was a time when colored leaves were everywhere around the island. That trip began with a music recital at Noburu's home in Tokyo. He and Jay sang the famous Elvis song, "Can't Help Falling in Love."

Discovering – and rediscovering – Indonesia

Jay has made eight trips to Indonesia and all of them involved spending time in Bali. When he first visited, he did not have any pre-existing knowledge about the country. "I never could have predicted the unusual experiences I would have in Indonesia over the course of several years. My travels there were a mini case study in *beshert.*"

His first trip to Indonesia came about because of a woman he met at a New York cocktail party in 1973. They talked about his upcoming around-the-world trip, with Stuart. The woman was originally from Indonesia and she insisted that Jay and Stuart go there as well. She said her family had strong ties to the United States – her father had served as the Indonesia's ambassador in Washington, DC – and that they would welcome Jay and Stuart if they could make time for a shortstop in Jakarta, Indonesia's capital city. "It would just be a very short detour to the south of your trip itinerary but worth seeing the island of Bali," she told Jay. "I know my father would be happy to meet you."

Jay and Stuart had never been to Indonesia and were intrigued by the offer to meet her father and her description of life in that large country. After traveling through Europe and India, Jay and Stuart flew to Jakarta in June 1973. They were told by the young woman from the cocktail party in New York that her father and other members of her family would meet them at the airport.

When they arrived, they saw hundreds of people waving white handkerchiefs, so they waved back and waited until someone approached them.

But no one did. And they didn't have phone numbers for anyone. "It was midnight, so we just spent the night on the floor of the airport," recalls Jay. "We thought the family would meet us in the morning."

Alas, no one showed, so they took a *tuk tuk* taxi to downtown Jakarta. Upon arriving there, Stuart went to a grocery store and bought some fruit. While waiting in line at the cashier, he struck up a conversation with a young woman and explained that they had hoped to meet the father of this young friend.

It was another *beshert* moment. The woman in front of him knew the family and lived nearby. She arranged for the boys to speak with the family. "We went to their home and realized that they'd had too many guests recommended by their daughter and they didn't want to entertain yet another guest," recalls Jay. "But they were very kind and gave us advice about our trip to Bali."

Jay and Stuart heard from the young woman about an elderly physician and his wife who lived nearby and enjoyed having guests stay with them. When Jay and Stuart met the couple, there was a strong connection. Their discussion eventually turned to art – an interest of both Jay and Stuart – and the couple told them about a family of artists whose name was Affandi. Their home was nearby and a museum was attached to it.

Jay and Stuart went to the museum and met the daughter of the museum's founder. Her name was Kartika and she showed them around the museum. They ended up buying some artwork by Kartika's husband, a prince from one of the country's tribes. That piece hangs in Jay's house today.

That encounter led to Jay, Stuart, and Kartika going out to paint together in the Jakarta region. It was the start of a strong bond with Kartika. "She became like a muse for me," recalls Jay, "and over the years she was always the impetus for a painting expedition."

Jay and Stuart flew to Bali the next day and stayed in small hotels that charged only one dollar per night. "We were there for five days and loved it," recalls Jay. "We met a lot of hippies wearing sarongs and we wore sarongs. We ate a lot of fresh fruit. We found this was a delightful, very attractive way of living."

During their next visit to Bali, two years later, they stayed at the Bali Beach Hotel, which was adjacent to a small beach. There they met an Indonesian couple who insisted that Jay and Stuart come visit them in their home region of Sumatra, a large island in western Indonesia.

Subsequently, when Jay and Stuart returned to Indonesia in 1974 they visited Sumatra and met with this couple from their previous visit. The husband was known as a *datuk*, which refers to someone with wealth and knowledge. During that visit, they were introduced to a foul-smelling fruit, known as a durian, which took time to appreciate.

The most memorable episode for Jay was a trip into a local forest. (The *datuk* didn't accompany them, but someone from the military did). It was an extremely hot day, so Jay and Stuart removed their shirts. When they did, they discovered that they were covered in land leeches, which had penetrated their skin. (Jay and Stuart had not noticed because the leeches secrete an anesthetic.) The leeches were removed by pouring salt on them.

After a few hours in the forest, it became clear to Jay and Stuart that their guide didn't know the way back to where they started. Fortunately, he had brought a gun, to fend off any attacks by animals. Soon after discharging the gun, some scouts materialized and showed the group how to get back to where they had their Jeep.

Jay was so enamored with Bali that he made it a stop on his honeymoon in 1977. He and Sharon flew in from Australia, and upon arrival at the airport they saw several people surrounding their small plane and greeted them. They wondered why there were so many people near their plane only to realize that Kartika and Stuart were dressed as a Prince and Princess in Indonesian costumes. The populace probably thought they were royal family. Music was playing, Kartika was in a traditional Indonesian wedding costume, and Stuart was in a traditional Balinese prince's suit.

"It was as if we were visiting royalty," recalls Jay. "It was one of the highlights of our honeymoon." A friend of Kartika hosted a wedding party for Jay and Sharon, which included a Balinese marriage ceremony. The couple owned two white puppies and Jay and Sharon carried them during the ceremony.

Playing the piano

Jay and Stuart asked for – and started taking – piano lessons when they were eight years old. They were taught weekly by Margery Hamilton Hill, who gave lessons to children from important society families in the Wilmington area. Hill taught classical music, but at 16 Jay stopped taking those lessons and focused his piano playing on popular music. "That made me more popular," recalls Jay, "as people wanted to hear popular songs. But at Wesleyan, all the piano players were much better than I, so I mostly stopped playing."

Jay resumed piano lessons in 1980, while living in San Francisco. There was a teacher from Japan named Kaiko, who lived just five blocks away from Jay and Sharon. The weekly lessons continued for about six years and the style was classical music. The last piece Kaiko gave Jay was a Rachmaninoff piece, "Prelude in C Sharp Minor." "I didn't need the sheet music," recalls Jay, "I remembered it from the past. My fingers remembered how to play the chords without much training. And to this day, I play it."

Jay once again returned to the piano when he was about 65 and played regularly for 3-4 years. He only stopped when he started experiencing back pain. "Music provided good balance for my life," he says. "It had a calming and uplifting effect on me. I was very disappointed when I couldn't sit straight, which is one of the ideal attributes for pianists."

Playing the ukulele

Stuart introduced Jay to the ukulele. Soon they were known as singing together with their strumming of the ukulele. Their repertoire was mostly folk songs, particularly those sung by the Highwaymen, who were fraternity brothers of Jay at Wesleyan. The boys recognized that these instruments were readily portable and could be a catalyst to get a group of people singing. Their favorite songs included 1960s staples such as "Cotton Fields," "Michael Row the Boat Ashore," and "We're on Our Way to Freedomland." "I played 'Freedomland' while in East Berlin. Me and my Wesleyan roommate, Mark Lischner, were several hours late returning to the border, which could have led us to be detained," recalls Jay. "But I played that song on the ukelele when we approached the guard station and the guards just waved us through."

Seeking the cause of chronic fatigue syndrome

During the time Jay was deeply involved in studies of AIDS, he also became interested in studies of patients with chronic fatigue syndrome (CFS). He was certain that it could stem from a virus and wanted to try to find the cause.

Jay's research indicated that CFS was due to an immune response activated by exposure to a variety of different infectious agents. But response to the infectious agent is often unsuccessful and the condition continues for many weeks and sometimes years. His research indicated that there are at least three markers of immune cell activation associated with this condition.[55]

He and his fellow researchers reported their finding in *The Lancet* in hopes that the discovery would be helpful to people with the condition. But it is difficult to calm down the immune system in a general manner without affecting the antimicrobial response. "A selective approach to reducing the activated response is needed," says Jay. "Quieting the entire immune system would permit other infections to develop."

He says that studies by others are needed to verify his observations, but that the concept is not unusual. "A variety of cells in the immune system react to an infection and my team has found that NK cells might selectively modify and reduce activation of these immune responses." He has suggested that the name of the condition be changed to "chronic immune activation syndrome," or CIAS.

Piero and Lucille Corti

During Jay's summer in Uganda, he worked at a well-known Catholic hospital in Gulu, St. Mary's Hospital Lacor. He had the good fortune to partner with two physicians who were married to each other, Piero and Lucille Corti (he was Italian and she was Canadian).

They would later become celebrated for the health-care services they provided, particularly for HIV-infected patients. Lucille performed more than 13,000 surgeries. But in 1985, she was diagnosed with AIDS, which she believed she contracted while operating on infected soldiers. As her health declined, medical professionals told her that she should seek treatment from a doctor in San Francisco.

That doctor was Jay. She showed up at his UCSF office one day, unannounced. She didn't realize he was the same person who had worked with her, more than 20 years earlier. "It was a great *beshert* moment," recalls Jay. "I immediately arranged for her to see a variety of physicians at San Francisco General Hospital," recalls Jay. "But there was not much we could suggest as treatment."

Lucille had only been given two years to live, but she survived until 1996 and continued to see patients until the very end of her life. She was buried on the grounds of the Lacor hospital and she was honored with several public ceremonies, one of which Jay and Sharon attended in Milan. A postage stamp was also issued in her honor, in Canada.

Jay knew the daughter of Piero and Lucille, Dominique, and she later became a physician in Montreal and helped to oversee a philanthropic foundation her parents had established in 1993, to support the Lacor hospital where they worked.

Addressing AIDS in Malawi

In 2018, Jay and Sharon visited Malawi, as part of Jay's involvement with the Global AIDS Interfaith Alliance (GAIA), a non-profit group focused on strengthening healthcare in underserved African communities. They met with government officials, physicians at the University of Malawi medical school, and with villagers served by GAIA.

"GAIA is revered and *highly* respected," says Jay. "The work being done by Joyce Jere, GAIA's country director in Malawi, and her team is remarkable and life-changing for thousands of people. They are bending the arc of an epidemic and doing so with kindness, smiles and love and one of the poorest regions of the world." (Since GAIA was founded in 2000, the prevalence of HIV in Malawi among people aged 15-49 has fallen from 15.3 percent to 6.2 percent.)

The visionary founders of GAIA, UCSF professors Bill Rankin and Charlie Wilson, wanted to bring health care and support to the far corners of Africa through programs involving the churches and religious activity in Africa. "What these two men lacked in knowledge of Africa and HIV they made up with their dynamism and empathy for this challenging pandemic," says Jay. "We were very impressed by the dedication to the country with beautiful tea plantations and pineapple groves." As a tribute to the two founders, Jay and Joyce planted two yellow flowering acacia plants in front of the GAIA office.

Sports

When Jay and Stuart had their bar mitzvah, Herb Steinberg, a friend of their father, gave them golf lessons, which were every Thursday evening at the YMHA. They supplemented the lessons by reading a very popular book at the time, *How to Play Your Best Golf All the Time.*

That summer, and for several that followed, they competed in the Delaware juniors golf tournament. They won the tournament a few times: "Stuart was much calmer and more focused than me" recalls Jay. Jay and Stuart also enjoyed swimming, particularly at the Brandywine Country Club in Wilmington. When they were eight years old and attending a summer camp in Pennsylvania, they surprised the camp counselors by swimming to an island a half mile away.

A classic car

When Jay was in Paris in 1960 on his Fulbright scholarship, he purchased a 1931 Citroen C4G for $150. The car did not have a key (it was started by pushing a button) and the turn signals were not up to code. He found a shop near Paris that addressed these issues, and one that repaired the antique Jaeger interior clock. Once it was in working order, it was one of the most noteworthy cars in Paris. He used it to climb Montmartre with friends, who stood on running boards on both sides of the car. Later, Jay drove the car to Le Havre, where it was shipped to San Francisco. Afterwards, he drove it for many years. But when it became too difficult to find a garage for it, he donated it to the Mullin Automotive Museum in Oxnard, California. (That museum is now closed and the cars are being distributed to other car museums.)

Language

Jay's history with foreign languages goes back to his four years of Latin in high school and his three years of French. His French greatly improved when living in France for nearly a year in between college and medical school. While living in Israel in the summer of 1962, he helped several immigrants in a small village near Jerusalem. He was given a room in the home of Jerusalem's mayor and was taught elementary Hebrew by the mayor's grandson, who was eight years old. But the lessons didn't last: "I stopped taking them from him when he laughed at me for mispronouncing the Hebrew word for 'excellent,'" recalls Jay. But he resumed the lessons with an Israeli at UCSF while living in San Francisco.

Jay also grew to appreciate Italian through his strong friendship with one his students, Tony Hoffman. When they first met, Tony's English was not very good and Jay suggested they meet regularly to speak in their native languages. Through several years of speaking Italian to each other and taking ski vacations in Italy, Jay became very comfortable speaking the language.

As noted earlier, before Jay went to Sweden in 1962 to work at the Karolinska Institute, he arranged to have a Columbia professor of anesthesiology from Sweden, Jan Gyessing, teach him Swedish. He thoroughly enjoyed speaking the language while living for two months in Stockholm.

A science camp

From 2007 through 2020, Jay was deeply involved with a science summer camp operated by UCSF. He often spoke about infectious disease and later about Covid. The camp targeted students who had just completed fifth or sixth grade, as science curiosity can be nurtured or lost at this age.

Students were exposed to hands-on science, UCSF students and faculty, and the UCSF Parnassus campus. Throughout the camp, in interactions with science and healthcare professionals, students were encouraged to pursue careers in natural and health sciences. Students who were of racial and ethnic minorities in science were targeted for camp enrollment, working to address underrepresentation in science and health professions.

The camp was the brainchild of a technician in Jay's lab, Heather Hertema. (She was also a student in the pharmacology department at the time.) In its first year, the camp attracted 60 students from schools in the Bay Area.

The experiments included dropping an egg from the roof of the health sciences building and selecting the student that had designed a case hoping to protect the egg. Also the best cardboard raft to cross the gym swimming pool. The students heard lectures on a wide range of topics, including biology, chemistry, and infectious diseases. The speakers included department chairs, professors, and the Chancellor.

Some of the students have gone on to teach science in high schools. In a great example of *beshert*, one of the students, Najwa Anasse, double majored in biology and neuroscience at Jay's alma mater, Wesleyan, and has since gone on to medical school in Cuba. "The UCSF science camp was the reason I became interested in science," she has said. "It was there that I held a real human brain in my hand, an experience that led to my fascination with neuroscience."[56] She worked in a lab focused on neuroscience and stem cell research, with an emphasis on stem cell therapy as a possible treatment for epilepsy.

Life lessons from painting

Jay's mother was an amateur painter but that wasn't what got him interested in it during junior high: "I tried hard to be selected to paint Halloween images on stores downtown because it got me 1) out of classes and 2) free time with friends."

The experience nonetheless lit a spark in him and he took a painting class his senior year at Wesleyan. He was given a key to the Davidson Arts Center, where he would sometimes go late at night "to paint as I felt." And he sometimes said that the painting course he took his senior year was a tutorial that included supplies. That ended up being a way to recover some of the tuition he paid. He later donated a painting of his childhood treehouse to Wesleyan's art collection.

While living in Washington, Jay discovered his enjoyment of putting oil paints and later acrylics into a painting. This expression of creativity came about because of a teacher in Chevy Chase, Maryland, a Washington suburb near the National Institutes of Health, where he was working at the time.

During his first night in the class, the teacher, Artie Ludwig, "passed by my painting and mistakenly thought my large green pasture was a large lake. She also commented that I must be a scientist because of the precision of my painting." She thus asked Jay to draw an apple in no more than 60 seconds (and used a stopwatch to measure the time). He did it, and that moment was an inflection point in his life. "I credit Artie with giving me the confidence to bring painting into my life," recalls Jay. "It has been a major part of my life ever since." Ludwig also brought in canvases of different shapes, to challenge Jay's artistry, and introduced him to painting techniques used by several different artists.

Later, she would challenge Jay to paint a range of shapes and images and add acrylic paint for a realistic scene (such as his carriage house in Georgetown). He also created fantasy paintings using canvas only and not with the stretcher. "By folding the canvas in different ways I was able to mimic veins," recalls Jay. "Running across large areas – painting them green gave them the look of blood circulation, even though red paint was not used. The result suggested a highly vascular organ like the placenta. Thus, the series had a name." Among his favorite paintings were renditions of skiers dwarfed in a mountain scene and a portrait of a sheepdog named Boris the Hungarian, who belonged to a close friend of his in Georgetown, Liz Verville.

A beshert *moment thanks to the FBI*

Another life lesson followed many years later. Jay was returning from a meeting of his lab colleagues at UCSF and his secretary, Kaylynn Peter, met him in the hallway. She warned him that there were two FBI agents in her office waiting to serve him a subpoena. The subpoena was an order to travel to Canada for a trial involving a hemophiliac patient infected by Factor VIII transfusion.

Kaylynn had the two agents wait in Jay's office and Jay returned to the conference room. After about 45 minutes, the agents warned Kaylynn that if she was helping Jay avoid them, she would be obstructing justice.

She told the agents that Jay was off campus but that she would relay the message to him. Jay decided to go home and the FBI agents told her that they knew he had a flight to Italy the next day.

Jay contacted the university lawyer, Cynthia Lynch, and she explained that there was an agreement between United States and Canada involving this kind of cooperation. She negotiated with the FBI agents and they reached an agreement that he would testify in California.

As this saga unfolded, the friend of an AIDS patient had been waiting to meet Jay in his office. She had noticed that his office was decorated with images he had painted. It turned out that she was the chair of a committee to select artists for the upcoming "Hearts in San Francisco" art campaign to raise money for San Francisco General Hospital. She invited him to submit a painted ceramic heart which was purchased for $15,000 in an auction held as part of the campaign. It was another *beshert* experience.

Chapter 13

Siblings in Science

On March 18, 2019, a research center at the Tufts University School of Medicine held a symposium devoted to fighting drug-resistant diseases. It was the school's first such symposium, which was named, "the Stuart B. Levy Tufts CIMAR Symposium." It was given than name, said Tufts, "to honor Dr. Levy, whose pioneering work in fighting antibiotic misuse and resistance was a key inspiration for CIMAR's inception."[57]

But Stuart was not the only Levy to have a prominent role that day. Jay also spoke, as did their sister, Ellen, a medical director of the Instituto Dominicano De Estudios Virologicos (IDEV) in Santo Domingo, Dominican Republic.

Jay spoke about lessons learned from antibiotics that could inform anti-HIV therapies, while Ellen spoke about the Alliance for the Prudent Use of Antibiotics (APUA), which Stuart founded and in which she was active. It is a global research and advocacy organization with 66 chapters and members in more than 100 countries.

The symposium was a testament to the achievements of three children from the same family. Two medical degrees and one doctorate – and all of them standouts in their respective fields – and emblematic of the family's commitment to advancing science and health, which started with their father's decades of work as a physician in the Wilmington area. This chapter focuses on the professional lives of Stuart and Ellen.

Stuart

Stuart attended Williams College, in Massachusetts, where he majored in English and graduated magna cum laude. He later attended medical school at the University of Pennsylvania. While there, he conducted research at the Pasteur Institute in France. He studied with Jay's scientific inspiration, Raymond Latarjet, who became a friend of the Levy family – yet another example of *beshert.*

In 1971, Stuart joined Tufts, as an assistant professor in the departments of medicine and microbiology. His first breakthrough study was published just a few years later. The study involved 300 chickens that had consumed tetracycline, an antibiotic used to make livestock grow faster, with their feed. He also took fecal samples from six families that were raising the chickens. He found that the stool samples of the chickens, and the families, contained a bacteria resistant to tetracycline.

"These data speak strongly against the unqualified and unlimited use of drug feeds in animal husbandry," he wrote with his two co-authors in a paper published in the *New England Journal of Medicine*, "and speak for reevaluation of this form of widespread treatment of animals."[58]

Stuart later called on the Food and Drug Administration to ban the use of antibiotics to stimulate growth in animals. He was strongly opposed by the agriculture and pharmaceutical industries. But one year before he retired from Tufts, the FDA introduced the ban. "The impetus and evidence that drove those policies goes back to Stuart's work," Dr. Helen Boucher, director of a fellowship focused on infectious diseases at Tufts Medical Center, told the *Wall Street Journal*. "That contribution cannot be overstated."[59]

Stuart had another breakthrough in 1978, when he co-authored a study showing that, as *The Lancet* put it, "Escherichia coli could evade the antibiotic tetracycline through the use of transport proteins called efflux pumps that dump the chemicals out of the microbes."[60] This "active efflux" mechanism "is now an accepted paradigm for a critical class of antibiotic resistance and is also a mechanism for resistance to drugs that treat cancer," noted Tufts in a tribute to Stuart shortly after his death.[61]

In 1981, Stuart founded a nonprofit group, the Alliance for the Prudent Use of Antibiotics. That year, nearly 150 scientists, representing 27 countries, issued a statement, under the umbrella of the APUA, about antibiotic misuse – generating stories in national newspapers and magazines, as well as scientific journals.

As the work of APUA continued, Stuart founded the Center for Adaptation Genetics and Drug Resistance at Tufts in 1992. And a few years later, he co-founded a company, Paratek Pharmaceuticals, with a Nobel laureate, Walter Gilbert. Paratek, which continues to operate, was focused on developing drug therapies for people with infectious diseases, with an early emphasis on research into how to overcome efflux pumps. The company's signature product has been a once-daily oral and intravenous antibiotic for the treatment of adults with community-acquired bacterial pneumonia and acute bacterial skin and skin structure infections.

In 2002, Stuart had a book published, *The Antibiotic Paradox: How the Misuse of Antibiotics Destroys Their Curative Powers.* A review published in the *New England Journal of Medicine* called it, "an accessible, fact-filled warning of the risks posed by the unwise use of the prize drugs – antibiotics. Nowhere else are the history of antibiotic discovery and the mechanisms of microbial resistance so clearly presented for general readers."[62]

A testament to Stuart's eminence in the field came a few years later, when the American Society of Microbiology published a 570-page book titled, *Frontiers in Antimicrobial Resistance: A Tribute to Stuart B. Levy.*[63] The book had 78 contributors (from 12 countries) – all of whom were authorities on antimicrobial resistance and students or collaborators of Stuart.

A Rutgers University microbiologist once said of Stuart, "For many years he was a voice in the wilderness, talking about things that were not a part of the conventional wisdom."[64] But Stuart made extraordinary progress, and in 2014 the World Health Organization called antibiotic resistance a "major threat to public health." A Harvard scientist told the *Washington Post,* for Stuart's obituary, that "It was Dr. Levy who catalyzed the transformation of antibiotic resistance into a shared, global concern, mandating global collaborations across various domains of medicine, science, industry, agriculture, and politics."

Stuart retired from Tufts in 2018 and passed away the following year, after a bout with Parkinson's. He is buried in Israel. Tufts published a tribute to Stuart, which included a quote by the chairman of the department where Stuart worked, John Leong. He described Stuart as "always extremely gracious, never dismissive. When I arrived in 2012 [as department chair], I asked him what role he'd like, what he needed. Stuart had only one request. He wanted to lecture first-year medical students and educate them on antimicrobial resistance. He didn't ask for more space or money. I thought that was remarkable."[65]

In September 2020, Tufts held a ceremony to celebrate Stuart and announced that the school's Center for Integrated Management of Antimicrobial Resistance was being named for Stuart.[66]

At the time of his death, Stuart was married to a dermatologist who had been born in France, Cecile Pastel. They had wed in 1984 and had three children: Suzanne, Arthur, and Walter.

Ellen

"Stuart and I enjoyed being twins," recalls Jay. "But we kind of felt sorry for Ellen during our childhoods, since she was three years younger than us and a bit removed from our everyday life, though we all bonded over our shared dislike of our housekeeper, Grace."

Even with the age difference, Ellen had much in common with Jay and Stuart. Like them, recalls Jay, "she was ambitious and wanted to be popular at school." She also participated in many of the same activities as Jay and Stuart. This included student government, playing sports (she was a standout tennis player – "unlike Stuart and me," says Jay), going to summer camp, and playing an instrument (the violin). She also chose to attend a small college in New England (Mount Holyoke). She earned a master's degree at the University of Pennsylvania, which is where Stuart attended medical school. She even continued some research that he had started during his student days.

During her time at Penn, she met a graduate student in economics, Mario Koenig, while they were both at one of the university's swimming pools. He had grown up in the Dominican Republic, though his parents were Holocaust survivors from Austria. They later married – at the Levy family home in Wilmington – and Ellen has lived in Santo Domingo for her entire professional life. "Here we educated our daughter at an eastern college," said Ruth (the mother of Ellen, Jay, and Stuart) in a conversation with Mario's mother, on the wedding day. "And she comes home with a guy from an island I've never heard of."

Like Jay, she has been focused on infectious disease – HIV/AIDS in particular. It was a fitting choice, given the prevalence of HIV/AIDS in the Dominican Republic. She and Jay were often pursuing research in similar areas and they collaborated on several papers. In 1987, they co-authored a letter to the *Journal of the American Medical Association*, focused on hepatitis B and HIV in the Dominican Republic.[67] She has also conducted research on cancer, autoimmune diseases, Covid-19, and viral infections.

Jay had recommended she research HIV/AIDS, which was a prompt for her to take blood samples from university students in the Dominican Republic. The samples showed that the virus had been present on the island since the early 1980s. When she started diagnosing people with HIV, she also wanted to be able to treat them. That led her to enroll in a local medical school, from which she graduated at age 50, with a medical degree.

Since then, she has remained focused on the study of viral diseases and public health in the Dominican Republic, through her affiliation with IDEV. She worked at the National Laboratory of Public Health, from 1995 to 1999, and she has helped future young scientists and public health professionals.

She has been honored for her work in public health and her innovative approaches to control of infectious diseases, which ranged from measles to mosquito-carrying arborviruses and COVID. She has been the go-to scientist for viral diseases in the Caribbean and helped establish and direct the Center for Viral Diseases, which is the leading virus institute in the Caribbean.

In 2010, Ellen was recognized by the president of the Dominican Republic, Leonel Fernández, for her achievements in science and technology. In 2015, she was named one of the women in the Dominican Republic who had delivered outstanding service to the country and its people.

Chapter 14

Conclusion

In 2023, Jay retired from UCSF, 53 years after he arrived. His pioneering work on HIV-AIDS strengthened the school's reputation as a first-rate academic medical center. His work lives on there (and beyond) through UCSF's AIDS Research Institute, which is focused on stimulating innovation and fostering collaboration across scientific disciplines. His work will also live on through the Jay A. Levy Endowed Professorship in Virology at UCSF. When seeking candidates, the school said it wanted someone embodying Jay's spirit as a researcher and mentor, with an emphasis on being "bold, innovative, with an impact both in the laboratory and beyond."[68]

Fittingly, the first person to hold the endowed professorship, Jeanette Tenthorey, has conducted research on HIV-AIDS. Much of her work is focused on what's known as "innate immune responses," which she characterizes as the "frontline response to infection, before your antibodies and your T cells really ramp up." She says she has studied HIV in particular "to try and understand if there might be 'evolutionary holes' in HIV, places in the evolutionary process where the innate immune system could find a foothold."[69]

She will carry on Jay's vital work against what was one of the world's deadliest conditions. It's fitting that his name is attached to a professorship that seeks candidates who have an impact beyond the lab, given that Jay has touched so many people who have no direct connection to science and research.

An endowed professorship is also fitting for someone who has spent virtually his entire adult life connected to academic institutions. And he has made scholarly contributions to two of them. In 2019, he donated to Wesleyan his personal correspondence with Samuel Beckett over nearly three decades. And late in his career at UCSF, he gave the university his lab notebooks, videotapes, cassettes, handwritten notes, posters, international correspondence and awards – approximately 140,000 pages of material.[70]

This material will advance scholarship, just as Jay has done with his teaching – both in the classroom (he taught classes in microbiology) and in his lab. He's proud of having mentored students and he says he's been heartened by those who have told him how much they learned from being around him.

One of the postdocs who worked in Jay's lab, Christopher Locher, wrote to him in 2025 and expressed gratitude for all of the knowledge he imparted. He singled out ten things:

> First, learn to write well. Then read what you wrote (out loud) and write it again, and again. Second, repeat experiments and do the proper statistics; biology is quantitative. Third, demand excellence from yourself first proactively. Fourth, do things right and do the right thing. Fifth, ask for help, don't be shy and when you do, speak up, louder. Sixth, willpower, just keep at it. Seventh, "you're going to have to give..." and care deeply and passionately about what you're doing. Eighth, type your notes right after a meeting along with the action items, circulate them to the team straight away. Ninth, keep your cell cultures healthy, use recombinant IL-2, and be mindful of the cell membranes (minimize cell death). Tenth, and most important, remember to live the values with unshakeable integrity, so your team will do so as well and bring out the best in

> themselves and others. Thank you for being a great role model for myself and for your scientists.

Jay viewed teaching as "a great part of medical training and a way to assess and challenge medical dogma." He would occasionally have students conduct experiments that had unexpected findings: "I wanted them to understand the important role that surprises in medicine can play in advancing our understanding of the human body."

That observation is a reminder that elements of Jay's life hold lessons for others. He has been willing to question conventional wisdom, which has opened avenues of exploration that can result in discoveries. An example is his contention that some cancers are created by the immune system. "Scientists – and everyone else – need to be open to ideas that are far out," he says.

As noted throughout the text, Jay also showed remarkable perseverance and resilience amid many challenges, particularly those at NIH and UCSF. While some researchers would have made noisy protests, and perhaps resigned, amid these challenges, Jay soldiered on. He credits the Weizmann Institute's Nechama Haran-Ghera with advising him not to get bogged down with critiques – or a lack of support – from higher-ups. "If you just handle your activities in the lab with integrity and answer the questions that have been asked of you, that is what is expected of a good scientist," she told him. The highest compliment, he says, would be for someone to tell him, "when the results are published by your group, I will believe them." Jay's ability to stay focused on what really mattered, and tune out the distractions, is a valuable lesson for anyone conducting research – but particularly those who are just getting started in the field and are destined to encounter obstacles.

Looking to the future of medical research, Jay says he is "optimistic" about the potential for artificial intelligence to "open up new knowledge in many different scientific disciplines, including virology." And he's heartened that institutions such as the Weizmann Institute remain dedicated to basic science, for the simple reason that "to make progress against any disease, you must have a deep understanding of the biological mechanism causing that disease."

Some have pointed out to Jay the apparent contradiction in an evidence-based scientist of his stature embracing a concept – *beshert* – that is grounded in a decidedly non-scientific idea: destiny. But Jay doesn't see any contradiction: "Scientists – and non-scientists, too – should be open to finding meaning in occurrences that don't have any logical explanation. Opening up your imagination contributes to your creativity, which can deliver great benefits."

Appendix 1

Befriending a Literary Lion

In 1992, Jay wrote an article about his interactions with the celebrated Irish playwright and poet, Samuel Beckett. The article, which appears here, was published by The American Scholar.

"This is like waiting for Godot," my friend said to me as we patiently waited at the Hartford airport for the arrival of my date for the big spring weekend.

With each hour that passed, her plane continued to be delayed. That comment, in 1959, led to my studies of Samuel Beckett and his famous play.

At Wesleyan University, I was a junior pre-medical student pursuing a dual major in French and biology. I had dedicated a great deal of time to studying the theater of the absurd as reflected by Camus, Sartre, Genêt, and Cocteau. Reading *Waiting for Godot* by Beckett, which was published only seven years earlier, initiated my longtime interest in this Irish playwright who was writing in Paris. It led to my senior thesis, "*Waiting for Godot,* Waiting for God?" From today's perspective, the title seems very simplistic. At the time, however, relatively little had been written about Beckett's play, and the idea that Godot stood for God, while suggested, was not well substantiated. Beckett made no allusion to it. A careful look through anthologies of the Bible and the Bible itself revealed what appeared to be direct analogies to biblical events in the play. In my opinion, the hypothesis of Godot as God was a plausible interpretation of this literary piece.

When I received Fulbright and French government fellowships to conduct biological research in Paris in 1960-61, my French professor at Wesleyan, Alex Szogyi, encouraged me to find Professor Mayou, head of French Studies at the Sorbonne, to show him my thesis. "Why not let him read your thoughts on Beckett?" he insisted. I waited eight months to do so. I suppose, reflecting on my stay in Paris, that a certain amount of timidity (not generally attributed to me) prevented me from contacting Professor Mayou sooner. Having received at least two letters from Professor Szogyi encouraging me, I finally telephoned Professor Mayou, who cordially received the call and asked that I leave my paper at his office. I waited several weeks to hear from him. Then one day I received a note at my hotel, Le Grand, on rue Dauphine, inviting me for drinks at his home. Our meeting, on a Thursday evening, April 18, 1961, was very pleasant and held in a typical French salon in the apartment. A canapé dominated the room where we sat and talked for almost an hour. He told me he enjoyed the paper and encouraged me to deliver it personally to Mr. Beckett at his apartment on boulevard St-Jacques. In fact, he said he had called Beckett to tell him that I might come.

Quite excited, I took the metro the next afternoon to an apartment building at 57 boulevard St-Jacques. As I was putting the manuscript into the mailbox in the lobby, Beckett arrived. I recognized him from a photograph I had seen in a book. Somewhat taken aback, I said to him in my best French that I had been sent by Professor Mayou, whom I assumed had already spoken with him. Mr. Beckett was extremely nice, and put me at ease despite his towering presence (I felt quite small at five foot seven inches next to his height of more than six feet). Beckett quickly mentioned that neither of us had to speak French (not our mother tongue), and we continued the formalities of our first meeting in English. In a warm but reserved manner he said he would get in touch with me after reading the paper.

In early June of 1961, I received a short note from Beckett inviting me to his apartment. He later gave me his private number to use in the morning between 11:00 A.M. and noon, the only time when he took phone calls. That number served as our means of communication for many years afterwards. I was very excited at his probable appreciation of my thesis, but I was also worried about how I should act upon meeting him.

Beckett, then fifty-six years old, received me at 5:00 P.M. on June 13 in the study of his apartment on the seventh floor of a relatively new building. He had been living there only six months. He was dressed casually in a green sports jacket, brown gabardine slacks, and a plaid tie. The room, full of books, had his wooden desk and some modern chairs. The walls were painted in pale yellow and light tan. His hair was turning gray, and again, from my vantage point, he was a tall, imposing gentleman, but with a soft voice. Almost immediately, he offered me a drink. "Be a nice change from Scotch," he said jokingly as he gave me a glass of Irish whiskey. We sat for more than an hour discussing his work, although in retrospect, probably in a somewhat superficial way. He asked me many questions about my life and my interest in biology. He shared with me his views on literature and assured me that he never denied that Godot was God; however, he did not intend it to have any specific meaning. Godot could be representative of one's goal or objective. He agreed that some of my analogies, such as the removal of shoes in the first act, fit biblical accounts about the respect given to holy places, but said that he in no way had the Bible in mind when he wrote the play.

During our conversation he told me how, at about my age (then I was twenty-two), he had met a writer, and later, because of the difficulty with that writer's sight, he was asked to be his scribe. At the time, I did not appreciate that Beckett was himself having eyesight problems, but I did appreciate the possibility that I was receiving an indirect invitation to join him as his assistant, as he had done for James Joyce. For a split second, I toyed with the fantasy of asking him whether he was looking for an assistant, but what would I answer to an affirmative reply? I realized that I had medical school and a science education ahead of me, and a father who did not even fully understand a year's interval from schooling. I decided, therefore, to consider this comment as merely a reflection on an event in his life that had some similarities to mine.

He told me how he loved the theater and saw it as truly representative of art, but hated when the performers played to the public: it ruined the play when they attempted to impress the audience. He mentioned that he particularly liked Dennis Johnson, who was Irish and the producer of several of his plays. He kept Beckett's lines exact—a feature Beckett demanded (although did not always get) from all directors of his plays. He said he had never tried cinema because he didn't know the medium. Nevertheless, some years later he would dramatically use this form of art in his short movie Film.

We discussed writers. He had never met Camus but respected him and enjoyed his work more than that of Sartre. Sartre he found too political in recent years. He thought Schehadé was very poetic – "an Oriental Parisien," but not dramatic enough despite good reading. He found Adamov "politically minded," whose early plays, particularly *Professor Taruma,* he liked best.

During our meeting, Beckett told me that he had just finished a new play called *Happy Days* and mailed it that morning to the publisher. No other comment about the work was made except that he wrote this play first in English and thought it would be produced in the States. He considered plays a rest from writing books. He gave me as a small gift *Comment C'est,* his latest book, and inscribed it. As I left he encouraged me to write him in August to plan another get-together before I left Paris. Unfortunately, since he was on vacation in late August and most of September, I did not have that opportunity before returning to medical school in New York.

By the time of our good-byes, he had already told me about his wife, Suzanne, whom I could hear in the kitchen adjoining the study. I would in later sessions ask to meet her, but never did. In other visits, I also subtly tried to get invited into other parts of the apartment, but, aside from one time in his kitchen, I was always greeted in his study, which changed little over the ten years I visited him there. In the following twenty years, we usually met at the Closerie de Lilas at Denfort-Rochereau and then later at the Café Francois at the PCM Hotel, which is located just across from his apartment on the boulevard St-Jacques.

In 1963, having seen *Happy Days* during one of its early performances in New York, I wrote Beckett a long letter about my enthusiasm for the show, for Ruth White, for the other performers, and for the excellent dialogue. When I purchased a copy of the play, I tried to locate the quotations that were part of the piece but found only a few that I could reference. During a subsequent visit to Paris, when we discussed this play in his study, I mentioned my interest in knowing how he had found these quotations. He told me that several came from old Irish writings and poems and promised to send me a copy of the play with the quotations cited. Several months later I received this well-annotated book, which has become a treasured part of my Beckett collection.

From July 1962 to June 1963, my twin brother, Stuart, also a medical student, spent a year in Paris working at the Institut Radium with Professor Raymond Latarjet. He, too, called Beckett at his special number and met him several times during that period. On several occasions, Beckett would call Stuart at his apartment on rue l'Abbé de l'Epée to arrange the meetings. One such get-together, on April 19, 1962, at the Closerie de Lilas, Stuart recalls as very cordial. It began with a tomato juice before they had lunch—piparade basque omelet. Their discussion included the theater, the cinema, and Beckett's reading of Edward Albee's play *Who's Afraid of Virginia Woolf?* Beckett preferred *Zoo Story* because it seemed better for the theater. Apparently, Alan Schneider had asked Beckett to translate *Virginia Woolf* into French, but Beckett thought it would not do well in Paris.

My brother Stuart asked Beckett how he decided to write. He replied, "When there was nothing else left for me to do ... I had no money, I started to write." He did not regard himself as a professional writer, but as a French "man of letters." "I write comme ca," he said. Stuart gave him several articles on science, but Beckett didn't have his glasses so it was difficult for him to read them. Nevertheless, showing a lot of charm and humility, he inquired about experiments in the laboratory. They were both amused by the interchange of their interests in science and the theater. Beckett offered an explanation. He said that the laboratory was like the theater. The scientist is the director and the test tubes are the players. "You may predict what will happen, but you do not know exactly how it is going to turn out."

My next visit with Beckett was on June 2, 1965, almost four years after our first meeting in Paris. Stuart and I met him at Closerie de Lilas for a delightful lunch. He was vigorous and lively, with more color in his face than I had remembered. His demeanor was once again warm and friendly. He was visibly pleased to see us together. We had drinks (our usual Irish whiskey) followed by the main course of salmon with salad. The lunch was topped by crepes suzette; he insisted we try them. We shared with him our recent trips to Africa in 1964 and our current research interest in tropical diseases. We were again touched by his enthusiasm for science and his knowledge of it. He told us of his new four-minute play *Va et Vient.* He joked that at first it was quite long, and he kept "perfecting" it. He translated it for a friend in England who was opening a cafe-theater and called the play *Come and Go.* According to Beckett, it did not translate well from the French. He also had written a short piece, *Eh Joe,* for the BBC. He told us of his visit to the States in July of the past year when he was working on a film directed by Alan Schneider. He did not want to go to New York but liked the challenge of doing cinema.

During that trip, his only visit to the United States, he entered the office of Grove Press and the secretary greeted him with the comment, "Mr. Beckett, it's a pleasure to see you here. I have 'hellos' from my two friends Stuart and Jay Levy." She was a friend of ours and forwarded our greeting on her own. He later graciously arranged for *Film*, starring Buster Keaton (his choice of actor for the role), to be shown to us whenever we would like. Needless to say, during the 1960s in medical school in New York, being able to call and have a private showing of a film by Samuel Beckett was nothing short of a "happening." I saw it before I left medical school for internship in Philadelphia. Stuart saw it when he came to New York for his post-medical training.

During that 1965 visit, Beckett also spoke to us of his wife's travels in Spain, Czechoslovakia, and Vienna with friends and their hopes of taking a month's vacation in August. He had a country home near Paris that he worked on when he could find the time. He shared with us as well his pleasure that his nephew, Edward, had won first prize in a flute composition at the Paris Conservatory. Edward was the son of his brother who had died from lung cancer. Despite this family tragedy, Beckett continued to chain-smoke throughout the years we knew him. He also spoke of his cousin's great ability in playing the piano. Both relatives were then in Paris and had been playing duets at his apartment for several days. Beckett loved music and greatly enjoyed these sessions.

Our conversation turned to golf and he mentioned that at one time his handicap was as low as seven. We invited him to visit us in the States where we could play the game together. He seemed genuinely interested in visiting, but said he had seldom played in the past thirty years. During this two-and-one- half-hour lunch, he also commented that Albee's play *Tiny Alice* was too long, and he understood why Sartre, for political reasons, refused the Nobel Prize in 1964. He was faithful to his belief, but Beckett questioned Sartre's refusal to accept an honorary degree from Columbia University since it was a private university.

During this reunion, Beckett also confided in us, who were now physicians, the problem of his failing eyesight. He told us that he was going to enter a nearby hospital, the Hotel Dieu, where the nuns would take care of him. Stuart and I inquired about this hospital and contacted other physicians in Paris to assure Beckett that his eye treatment was the best available. His poor eyesight was present during the making of his film in New York, and clearly its relevance to the film was apparent: the emphasis on the eye is paramount to the theme. (He was operated on for cataracts in 1970 and 1971.)

My next meeting with Sam (as he now signed his letters) was July 27, 1971, ten years after our first conversation. We met at the Closerie. Dressed in a brown sports coat, tan pants, and a dark blue tie, he was as warm and genuine as ever and acted as if we had not been long separated. He would not discuss the Nobel Prize awarded two years earlier. He spoke about his eye surgery, about which he had written me in March of that year. The first cataract was removed in October 1970 and the second in February of this year. "Both were successful and close vision is excellent." Sam had wanted the operations done near home in case he wandered and could not easily find his way back to the apartment. He didn't feel he would like contacts and was surprised to learn that I wore them. I took one out to show him. He seemed interested and said he might try them.

We talked of his father in Ireland who was a surveyor—"a boring job"—and of his older brother (by four years) who "unfortunately took the same profession." He was the one who died in the 1950s from lung cancer. Beckett refused to believe cigarette smoking was involved in the cancer, and he remained a chain-smoker. In 1968, Beckett had lung abscesses and stopped smoking for one year but then took it up again. We talked also this visit about his uncle, his last living relative, who had died a few months earlier. Apparently he had had poor circulation and had lost both legs and then went blind—almost like the character from *End Game*. Still the man remained quite happy, active, and alert. Sam seemed impressed with this. I asked him whether this uncle was the basis for the character in *End Game*, but he said he had written the play before his uncle's illness.

Beckett mentioned that he had last visited Ireland in 1968 when he went home for the funeral of his beloved aunt. He said he wouldn't go again because of what he feared would be too much publicity. Some years earlier, Beckett told me, he had taught two years in France and a few years at Trinity College in Ireland, but he didn't like it. This time he said he truly wanted to be a teacher but didn't admit it because now he'd be a professor at Trinity. He preferred to write and had decided that was the profession to follow. During this visit in 1971, Sam also told me how he became associated with the rather controversial production *Oh, Calcutta!* He was asked to write a script for the show and thought it would be a vaudeville-like review and contributions would be anonymous. At this visit he called it "rubbish." In his original writing of this thirty-second piece called *Breath*, a baby cries in the center of the stage, the light goes up with the cry, then descends and then another cry occurs. The producer changed it and added naked bodies to the performance. He was angered but was only able to get his name disassociated with productions outside the United States.

We spoke of Suzanne, who he mentioned loved Italy where they had just been on vacation. Beckett smiled with real affection when he talked of her. She used to teach as well. When we parted, I noted that he was now wearing gold-rimmed, regular glasses, not the dark bifocals. He was thinner than before but looking about the same after six years.

Our next meeting was December 16, 1971. I met him at 5:30 in the afternoon at his apartment. I remembered the entrance and mailbox where I had left the paper more than ten years before. He met me at the elevator on the seventh floor. He had a slight cold but otherwise was much the same. He wore tan slacks and a maroon turtleneck. He took me around the office area where I had been before. I saw paintings over his couch; the walls were cracking with age, and lots of books were scattered behind his desk. I gave him a copy of the chimpanzee article that Stuart and I had published in *Nature* after our trip in 1970 to find human viruses in this primate species in Africa. He seemed touched that I had thought of bringing it. He said that he had spent most of his time recently working on new prose. He had no plays in mind at the moment. I asked him if he felt as enthusiastic and energetic as he did ten years ago or whether he was ready to relax. He said, with a smile, "No, I still have a lot of spunk left in me if that's what you mean." He was eager to get back to writing now that his eyes were better, and he was happy that he could drive again. He enjoyed going to his country home about forty-five minutes by train from Paris, where he would pick up his old car and drive to the house. It was a small place with a bedroom, kitchen, and dining room, on about one hectare of land. He had done a lot of his writing there over the past ten years.

I ventured to ask him what he considered his best play and was surprised when he answered *End Game,* not *Waiting for Godot.* He couldn't give details on why he felt this way. We walked into the kitchen to get ice for our Irish whiskeys. From the windows, since it was clear outside, I could see many rooftops of Paris, and it reminded me of the view I had had from my fifth-floor walk-up at Le Grand Hotel in 1961. Before he had moved to this apartment in the fifteenth arrondissement, he had lived with Suzanne in an apartment nearby. When asked about his family, he said he had very few family members in France aside from a cousin, a social worker in a nearby hospital. When I left after three hours, it was only because I was late for dinner with friends. Beckett asked me to call him in January before he went south to Morocco to find "some sun," but we were unable to arrange another meeting that year.

In 1976, Stuart again spent several months doing research in Paris at the Pasteur Institute. He took the occasion to meet Beckett, usually at his apartment. Stuart again shared results of his laboratory experiments with Sam and was encouraged by his enthusiasm for the work. In June of that year, Stuart asked Sam if he would meet our parents during the time of their visit to Paris. Much to his surprise, Sam said that he would be very pleased and accepted Stuart's invitation to come to his apartment to have cocktails with them. My mother's remark, "What will I say, I've never met a real intellectual" has become legendary in the family. But the man they met proved to be no intimidating figure. He had walked from his apartment on boulevard St-Jacques to visit them at 4 rue du Four—about a twenty-minute walk. He strode into the room, relaxed in a wide-winged chair, and proceeded to carry on casual conversation, including a discussion with my father about his early days playing golf in Ireland. At that time, Beckett had scored in the high seventies. They all had drinks and talked about many different subjects of common interest. He showed Dad, a physician, his right hand with the Dupuytren's contracture. The shortening and thickening of the tendons in the palm had caused a deformity of his index finger.

Beckett was not in a rush and stayed about two hours. Thus, to our family, Samuel Beckett was certainly not the recluse often cited in comments about him and his life. In all our relationships with him, he was always a warm, receptive, and generous man. Over the years, he shared with me several texts that he wrote, and he answered all of my letters, if just by a small note, including our last exchange about six months before his death. One treasured volume he sent in 1977 to my wife, Sharon, and me as a wedding gift—one of the first printings of his book on Proust *(Three Dialogues)*.

It was, however, two years after that, in 1978, when I would meet him again. This time, we got together at the Café Français at the PCM Hotel at 17 boulevard St-Jacques just across the street from his hotel. We met there because he said the tourists bothered him now at the Closerie. He arrived at about 11:00 in the morning. You could see him walking in his characteristic lanky manner, a little more unsteady than before. Sharon was with me at the time; we were on our way for a sabbatical year, the first half in Israel and then the second half in Paris. He began by inquiring about Stuart and our parents and asked about my research. As I was discussing it in some detail, he turned to Sharon and said, "Jay always thinks I understand what he's doing, but I just look like I do." He asked as well about the study Stuart had done on the transfer of bacterial antibiotic resistance from chickens to man. Despite his earlier comment on his limited knowledge of science, I was still amazed at how much he understood and that he remembered details from our previous conversations.

This time Beckett talked again about his trips to Germany to direct some of his plays. He traveled there every other year, and recently had met Jack Kerouac. He also went to Morocco for "some sun and swimming," and he was now translating and not working on anything new. I dared to ask him about his impressions of the biography of him by Deirdre Bair. He quickly remarked that he didn't want to talk about it: "I threw it away." Knowing he guarded his privacy, I was not surprised. We discussed Albee, who was supposed to be writing a new play. Beckett said that his problem was directing his own plays. That was a curious remark since Beckett was doing the same. We also spoke of Alan Schneider and how I had had the pleasure of being with him at Stanford for a three-day course on Beckett. Sam liked him very much because Schneider directed his plays correctly.

Beckett would, from time to time, engross me in conversations about my research in France or in the United States. When I first met him in 1961, I was working with Professor Lender at the Faculté de Science in Orsay on regeneration of planaria. When this freshwater flatworm is cut in half, it regenerates its tail or its head, whichever is missing. I kept thinking that Beckett might use this biologic event as some theme for a future literary piece of the "absurd"—but he never surprised me with that. Our discussions on cancer, and later on AIDS, always reflected his great interest in the subjects and his concern for finding solutions to these human diseases. But, most of all, I appreciated Sam's remembering certain details of my scientific work that I had discussed with him even years before. He was able to conceptualize areas of scientific study and to ask provocative questions.

Nine months later, after our return to Paris from Israel, Sharon, Stuart, and I met Beckett again at the Café Français. He looked healthy, active, and happy to see us. He recounted that he began playing golf at the age of twelve or thirteen and played with his Uncle Girard, a doctor, and his cousin. He commented that he knew Sartre in school in Paris. The man was "famous for his practical jokes; some of them cruel-like telling the professor his daughter had died in a car accident." He didn't know Simone de Beauvoir and never had met Gertrude Stein. She apparently had had a group of protégés separate from the one that surrounded James Joyce. He said similar literary associations exist in Paris today but are less defined and, in any case, he was not in any of them.

He had spent some time in January of that year in Tangiers with Suzanne in a hotel near the beach. He loved it there. He was going to his country home near Paris later in March and then on to London at the end of April to direct *Happy Days*. When we left we asked if we could take a picture. He graciously agreed, and Sharon snapped one of us with Sam, braced against a strong wind.

On April 20, 1980, Beckett wrote me, "Thank you for your letter of April 7 and your interesting account of *Piece of Monologue* at Stanford. Piece because unfinished—not to be continued. Light, walk, etc. have no symbolic significance for me. Dramatic components, nothing more." And, in a letter in July 1981, he wrote, "I had nothing to do with the staging of *Premier Amour*. The permission was for a straight reading. I have given no permission for staging Godot. So it goes in the theater."

I didn't see Sam again until June 26, 1986, during the time of the International AIDS meeting in Paris. My sister Ellen and I met him at the Café Français. We saw him standing in the lobby by the front desk looking out at the street. He was still impressive, though bent over a bit, and somewhat thin and frail. It was 11:00 A.M., our usual time to get together. Sam had never met Ellen, and I was eager to introduce him to yet another member of the family. He walked with a limp and seemed a bit weak, although his steel-blue eyes were still quite impressive. He showed me again his deformed right finger with Dupuytren's contracture. He complained of his breathing, but that difficulty had somewhat improved with time. He said he was in the hospital with emphysema—obviously from his smoking. He had just gotten out ten days before and felt better because he now used a spray. I again lectured him on cigarettes, but he said he smoked only ten a day. He asked, as usual, about my parents, Stuart, and Sharon. His speech was somewhat deliberate, and his mind, at eighty-one, seemed to be working at a slower pace.

He reminisced a bit about Sylvia Beach and her bookstore. He remarked that he had never read *A Moveable Feast* by Hemingway but told me not to send it, since he was trying to get rid of things around him. He lamented that Suzanne had cataracts, which had been operated on two months earlier, but she was doing all right. When he spoke of her, he seemed sad as if aging were more of a concern than before. He recalled his eye operations and the initial poor accommodation of his sight, although now his eyes were fine.

Despite his success and the fact that his publisher was good to him, I was surprised to hear that he had no secretary. He said he was not writing anything because of his constant lung problems and weakness—"just fixing up my affairs." He had hoped to go to the country where he kept his twenty-year-old car ("rusty but it works"). He was working on *Ohio*

Impromptu. One interesting point he made at that meeting came when he reminisced about his concern about *Film.* At one point he had wanted the camera to focus on Buster Keaton's eyes, both close up and far away without any realization of change, but it didn't work because the lens was not good enough. He walked us to the corner and said good-bye as we went to the metro. In his usual manner, he checked to be sure we knew how to take the train.

In October 1988, Sam sent me a note stating, "Thank you for yours of October 3rd with good news of your research in pursuit of that scourge. Nothing of interest to tell. Age has clawed me in his clutch. Affectionately to you all, Sam." I found it interesting that he referred to age in the masculine gender.

My last communication from him came in June 1989, when Sharon and I were in Paris for a meeting. We had hoped to see him again and his short note to me at the Mayflower Hotel read, "I am in a maison de retraite with health problems and cannot propose a meeting. Very sorry to miss you. Best wishes to you all. Sam." I regret now that I did not try harder to see him, for he died some months later.

During my several conversations with Samuel Beckett, he told me how very important it was that his plays be produced and directed in the way that he intended. He thought that the late Alan Schneider was the best director for his plays and had no problems in sharing any new works with him. These discussions on the direction of his plays led to his complaining to me during our first meeting, in 1961, about a rendition of *Waiting for Godot* about to be performed in Scotland; he had hoped to block it by legal action. "The production was billed as a rollicking comedy." He was appalled by the writer's changing of his intentions and "cheapening" the literary sense of the play. For example, he said to me, "Rien à faire," the opening line that in French means "nothing to be done," was loosely interpreted for the play as "nothing's doing." Subsequent lines also gave evidence to this "vulgarisation" of his French version. It was also at this time that Beckett said to me, with a twinkle in his eye, that *Waiting for Godot* told the audience from the very start what was going to happen in the next three hours—"nothing."

In discussions with my brother Stuart, Sam confided that one of the reasons James Joyce held back his friendship from Beckett was Joyce's disappointment that he did not marry his daughter, Lucia. While this point has been made in some books about Beckett, we were touched that Beckett shared this information with us and substantiated some of the stories that later appeared in his biographies.

One basic characteristic of Samuel Beckett was his deep humility. On one visit, when I congratulated him upon receiving the French Book Award, he insisted that we change the subject. He told me that he did not like awards or the attention they brought him. Subsequently, when he won the Nobel Prize in 1969, Stuart and I telegrammed him from Washington, D.C., where we were doing research at the National Institutes of Health. The telegram arrived in Paris and was forwarded to him in Tunisia where he was vacationing (or avoiding the publicity). Shortly thereafter we received a letter of thanks from him for the telegram, but subsequent reference to his Nobel award would also be cut off by his changing the subject.

Some of our conversations over those nearly thirty years dealt with issues I felt Beckett might not like to speak about with others. I was neither a writer nor a scholar doing re- search on his works. Instead I was a twenty-two-year-old pre-med student when we met, and our friendship continued because we shared a love of the theater and of French, and because I admired Beckett's challenging literary pieces. Sam saw me in a different field of study—medicine—and in many ways followed my career's development and the evolution of my family with a warm interest. During our last meeting in Paris I spoke to him, with a sincerity that I was never quite sure he fully appreciated, of the faith and optimism I drew from his experiences—particularly the problem he faced in publishing *Waiting for Godot*. I often share that story with my students and scientific colleagues who have their papers, grants, or books rejected. Samuel Beckett sent *Waiting for Godot* to many different editors, and it was finally accepted after four years by a small publishing company. The rest is history.

Appendix 2

Correspondence with the Nobel Committee

Nobelkommittén för fysiologi eller medicin
The Nobel Committee for Physiology or Medicine

December 17, 2007

Professor Jay A Levy
Department of Medicine
University of California, San Francisco
513 Parnassus, Room S1280
San Francisco, CA 94143-1270
USA

Dear Professor Levy,

We are very grateful to you for agreeing to write an evaluation on the role of clinicians in contributing to the concepts on AIDS that led to the discovery of HIV. A brief clarification of the evidence upon which you base your view would be most helpful. In the case of a positive view we would also be grateful for any name suggestions.

Your evaluation and all material pertaining to it are obviously confidential. Excerpts from the code of statutes for the Nobel Foundation are included in this letter. You will obtain a remuneration. We would be grateful if your evaluation could reach us by February 1, 2008.

If you have any questions or concern pertaining to this matter, please do not hesitate to contact me. My office number is +46-8-524 87802, mobile +46-70-570 3071 and my home number +46-8-34 05 15. Please do not use fax or e-mail in this matter.

With my best wishes,
Sincerely yours,

Hans Jörnvall
Secretary of the Nobel Committee

UNIVERSITY OF CALIFORNIA, SAN FRANCISCO

BERKELEY • DAVIS • IRVINE • LOS ANGELES • MERCED • RIVERSIDE • SAN DIEGO • SAN FRANCISCO SANTA BARBARA • SANTA CRUZ

DEPARTMENT OF MEDICINE
DIVISION OF HEMATOLOGY/ONCOLOGY
SAN FRANCISCO, CALIFORNIA 94143-1270

TEL: (415) 476-4071
FAX: (415) 476-8365

February 25, 2008

Mr. Hans Jörnvall
Secretary of the Nobel Committee
The Nobel Assembly
Box 270
SE-171 77 Stockholm
Sweden

Dear Mr. Jörnvall,

Enclosed is my commentary on the role of clinicians in the identification of AIDS and the discovery of HIV. I regret my delay in returning it to you, but hope my comments are helpful. If I can be of any other assistance, please let me know.

With kind regards,

Jay A. Levy, M.D.
Professor of Medicine

Enc.

JAL/kp

Comments on the Recognition of AIDS and Discovery of HIV

As you requested, I will share with you the early events that led to our recognition of AIDS in the San Francisco Bay Area, and the discovery of HIV. You have asked that I particularly concentrate on clinicians who helped identify AIDS as a new disease entity. Among those I would list Michael Gottlieb, Fred Siegal, Alvin Friedman-Kien, Donna Mildvan, Henry Masur, and Willy Rozenbaum. Details on their contributions can be provided by others.

In the Bay Area, the physician who first brought what we now call AIDS to our attention was Marcus Conant. Marc, a practicing dermatologist, had been in communication with Alvin Friedman-Kien in New York and alerted my former postdoctoral fellow, Paul Volberding, in 1981 about this new clinical entity. Paul had just left my laboratory to assume the position of Head of Oncology at San Francisco General Hospital (SFGH). Paul called me in August 1981 and asked me to discuss, during Medical Grand Rounds at SFGH, an unusual case of Kaposi's sarcoma in a young homosexual man. Donald Abrams was the oncology fellow who presented the case. I discussed the possible viral etiology of Kaposi's sarcoma (KS) and referred to my experiences in Uganda in 1964, when I was studying Burkitt's lymphoma. I interacted there with the Giraldos who had observed herpesvirus-like particles, suspected to be cytomegalovirus (CMV), in KS lesions. In my discussion at SFGH, I reminded the physicians and students that transforming DNA viruses would normally not replicate in cells that they transform since cell death would result. That might not be true for RNA viruses. In this case of KS, I raised the possibility of a herpesvirus being involved, which I predicted would be in an integrated or latent state, and producing transforming proteins leading to malignancy.

At the time, the patient, Dan Turner, was being followed by Marc Conant. Subsequently, Marc arranged for me to get some skin biopsy specimens from Mr. Turner and I began the first experiments in 1981 culturing KS lesions to find the KS virus. I worked in a small 80 sq. ft. laboratory which had been established for me to conduct human cancer virus research. In those days we were also required even within that space, to have a small anteroom to change into gowns and to double glove before working with human specimens. This work resulted in several KS-derived cell lines.

Shortly after I began the KS studies in 1981, I became aware, based on the work of Michael Gottlieb and the other clinicians, that CD4+ cell numbers were reduced in the subjects with KS and *Pneumocystis jiroveci (carinii)* pneumonia, reflecting an immune deficiency. It appeared that CD4+ cell destruction was the major cause of the disease syndrome. At that time, this condition became known as the gay-related immune deficiency syndrome or GRID. It took another year (1982) before it was called the acquired immune deficiency syndrome (AIDS). In San Francisco, we were aware then that similar clinical cases had been observed in Los Angeles, New York, Atlanta, New Orleans, and Miami (particularly among Haitians).

Marc Conant established a Kaposi's sarcoma clinic and discussion group at UCSF which had meetings on a regular basis during 1981-1983 at which many of us spoke and discussed various features of AIDS. I, for instance, gave an overview on different viruses that might be involved and concluded that GRID/AIDS was caused by a new agent and not a variant of CMV, Epstein-Barr virus (EBV), hepatitis B virus, or another known virus. In contrast, Larry Drew, at

1

Mt. Zion Hospital, felt AIDS resulted from an infection with a CMV-related or EBV-related virus. The search for a viral etiology of AIDS began then in San Francisco with my laboratory taking on the challenge of finding a new virus and the Drew laboratory looking at CMV and EBV.

Unfortunately, the University felt that the biosafety hood that we were using in my laboratory for our studies was not up to standard, and we were required to buy a new filter that cost $1500. In 1981, the Reagan administration had cut back dramatically the federal funding for research and I was unable to find the money to modify the hood. Through the help of Marc Conant, we finally obtained the funds from the California legislature, and began in 1983 to culture peripheral blood samples from AIDS patients.

In 1983, as a physician at UCSF, I was able to obtain blood specimens from patients, either who called me directly or were referred to me by Drs. Volberding or Conant, and other infectious disease doctors in San Francisco. Full evaluation of these specimens, using separated peripheral blood mononuclear cells (PBMC) placed in culture, was limited because my laboratory did not have a centrifuge to spin down culture fluids to look for a variety of viruses, particularly retroviruses. When Willie Brown, the Speaker of the House in the California legislature, decided to address AIDS as a major focus of attention in California, he invited those of us working in this field to Los Angeles to help draft a request for funds from the State of California. Thus, at 5:00 AM one morning in early 1983, Art Ammann, Murray Gardner, John Greenspan, Dan Stiles, Paul Volberding, John Zeigler, and I flew down to Los Angeles to begin working that morning on a request for funding from the State legislature. I was Chair of the virology section; Richard Gaynor from UCLA was my assistant. At the end of the session that afternoon, when the Speaker came in to thank us, we had arrived at a budget of $2.9 million.

That budget was approved by the State legislature in May 1983, but the Dean of the UCSF Medical School would not allow any of us to receive the funds. Only with intense negotiation, did my laboratory finally obtain some funding ($50,000) so that we could purchase an ultracentrifuge (September 1983) for our viral studies.

Back in April 1983, I read with interest in *Science* about the isolation of a retrovirus from a lymphadenopathy patient by the Pasteur Institute group. In the same issue was a paper by the NIH group describing the recovery of the human T-cell leukemia virus (HTLV) from AIDS patients. The conclusion of two papers was that HTLV or a variant of the virus had been isolated (1, 2). My first reaction was enthusiasm for the French group since I had worked with some of them and knew Luc Montagnier during my 1979 sabbatical in Paris. I was pleased that the Pasteur group had been able to isolate a virus from a lymphadenopathy patient but did not share their conclusion that a virus related to HTLV could cause AIDS. I discussed this point widely and was criticized by Robert Gallo at meetings and in the press for not accepting HTLV as the etiologic agent of AIDS. I reasoned that HTLV could not cause AIDS since it is too cell-associated, not cytopathic for CD4+ cells (but transformed them), and, thus, could not be spread by the means cited in the early epidemiological studies of AIDS: intimate sexual contact, contaminated blood (e.g. intravenous drug use), and, later, mother-to-child transmission. Notably, the work of the epidemiologists was very helpful in defining the risks for this disease and, thus, the type of agent that might be involved.

In October 1983, I attended the wedding of my twin brother, Stuart, to a French physician in Paris. At the time, I visited the Montagnier laboratory on a Saturday morning to say hello and to congratulate them on their work in the field. I was still not convinced that the Pasteur group had found the cause of AIDS since their agent was described as an HTLV-related virus. In addition, at an international immunology meeting in Japan in July 1983, one of their associates, probably Marc Alizon, had discussed the isolation of the virus by the Pasteur group, but had said that the serology showed antiviral antibodies only in French sera. Several of the attendees concluded that this was an agent only present in France, and thus could not be the universal cause of AIDS or related diseases. During this visit in France, I learned more about the Pasteur agent called LAV and, particularly, its cytopathology. I felt that if it were the cause of AIDS, it should be found in AIDS cases elsewhere, especially in San Francisco.

On my return to the United States, my laboratory was now equipped to look for the cause of AIDS with a certified biosafety hood and an ultracentrifuge. Within a month, we began detecting reverse transcriptase activity in the fluids of cultured PBMC from patients with AIDS. We began calling these agents AIDS-associated retroviruses (ARV) and numbered them sequentially following their isolation from the PBMC cultures. High levels of reverse transcriptase activity were detected, particularly with our second isolate, ARV-2. That virus, cultured to high titers in fresh peripheral white cells, was sent to my colleague (in murine leukemia virus research), Lyndon Oshiro, for electron microscopic evaluation. He confirmed the presence of a retrovirus. At that time my laboratory was very limited in personnel because of the cutbacks in funding. I did have a young college student, Tony Hoffman, who took on the task of perfecting the quantification of virus through reverse transcriptase measurements (3). All the culturing of the PBMC and bone marrow specimens and the cell culture studies were done by myself or my technicians.

In November 1983, my laboratory had identified the presence of retroviruses in several blood specimens, but not in all AIDS patients, patients with lymphadenopathy syndrome, or people from the known risk groups. Parenthetically, it was at that time that I had lunch with Peter Duesberg and told him of our work on the isolation of a retrovirus. Because we could not find the virus in every instance, Peter apparently concluded that it could not be involved in this disease. He did not appreciate that the techniques we used in culturing PBMC would not avoid the activity of CD8+ lymphocytes, which we later found had an anti-HIV inhibitory response that limits the isolation of the virus (see below).

Based on my past experience with immunoflourescence assays working with Gertrude and Werner Henle on EBV (4), I also quickly established an immunoflourescence (IFA) assay to detect seurm antibodies to the retroviruses we were finding in the PBMC of AIDS patients and people at risk for AIDS. Larry Kaminsky, a fellow in dermatology, joined the laboratory to learn virology and he became an expert in these IFA assays (5). He could obtain a result in 20 minutes and, for a period of time we were providing informal information on serum anti-ARV antibodies to our clinical colleagues, the renal transplant services, the San Francisco City Clinic, and to the San Francisco blood bank. We shared our IFA assay with the City Clinic and with other laboratories in San Francisco during 1984 and this procedure was established as a means of finding ARVs before the ELISA for HIV was developed.

3

One of the perplexing issues that made me hesitant to conclude definitively that a retrovirus was the cause of AIDS was the observation that hemophiliacs were developing this syndrome. When I inquired of Bruce Evatt whether all the affected hemophiliacs also had received a blood transfusion (the most likely source of a transmitted agent), he replied that some subjects had <u>only</u> been treated with Factor VIII. Thus, I questioned whether a retrovirus would survive the procedures involved in preparing Factor VIII and Factor IX.

To evaluate this possibility, I contacted, in November 1983, five different blood product companies in the California area and one, Cutter Laboratories, was willing to work with us. Because of my past experience with mouse xenotropic (X-tropic) retroviruses, we chose to use a particular X-tropic isolate that grew to very high titer (10^8 infectious particles/ml), to spike human plasma and follow the infectious virus titer through various procedures. That work indicated to us in March 1984 (6), that infectious retroviruses could survive the clotting factor preparation procedures. I then became much more convinced that the ARVs could be definitely linked to AIDS in all populations known to be at risk for the syndrome.

That month, I was invited to a meeting on HTLV in Washington organized by Robert Gallo. I was instructed that we would not be discussing AIDS, but only HTLV. At the meeting, however, there were some side comments concerning certain major findings on a retrovirus associated with AIDS and I initially presumed it was again the HTLV reported by the NIH and the Pasteur groups in 1983. With our findings on clotting factors, I wrote up our results on ARVs and sent the paper at the end of May to *Science*. I had also discussed our observations on the association of ARVs with AIDS early that month at the annual meeting of the American Association for Cancer Research (AACR) in Toronto. That same month in *Science*, the papers from the Gallo laboratory appeared connecting an HTLV-III to AIDS (7-10). Notably, our results, published in *Science* two months later (11), definitely showed in AIDS patients and others from known risk groups the presence of a cytopathic retrovirus that was different from HTLV and appeared to be somewhat different from the virus isolated by the Pasteur group. Françoise Barré-Sinoussi had provided me with fixed cells infected with LAV and we did not get a consistent reaction with those cells by IFA using San Francisco anti-ARV sera (11). We later concluded that our findings with LAV may have shown the diversity in HIV isolates that was only later appreciated.

This latter important observation on viral heterogeneity, not expected apparently by the NIH group, was eventually emphasized by Murray Gardner's group when comparing LAV, HTLV-III and ARV (12). That information, which identified HTLV-III as LAV, indicated that ARV was a totally separate isolate. In fact, when I presented our findings to Malcolm Martin's group at the NIH in probably August 1984, he advised me to be careful since our agent was so different from LAV and HTLV-III. I explained to him that, by molecular analysis, all our isolates were different (13). Martin's sudden realization of this important fact led to his recognition that HTLV-III was actually LAV that had been sent from the Pasteur group to the Gallo laboratory. Our ARVs were identified without any materials provided by the Pasteur group and they represented several different isolates.

Importantly, our 1984 publication presented the totally independent isolation of retroviruses from AIDS patients as well as other groups found to be at risk for this clinical syndrome. Because our agents were cytopathic and did not cross-react serologically with HTLV, we concluded that these were new human retroviruses with characteristics more like LAV than HTLV. Thus, this type of virus, originally detected in a lymphadenopathy patient, was now found to be associated with AIDS and in individuals outside of France. In this one article, antibodies to ARVs were also reported to be found in all populations at risk for AIDS and notably healthy subjects. This latter finding indicated for the first time, an asymptomatic carrier state.

This latter observation led to our pioneer work studying HIV-infected individuals who have remained healthy with normal CD4+ cell counts for a long time (in the early days, 1 year; and now, over 10 years) whom we identified as "long-term survivors." (Some have since called these people "long-term non-progressors.") Studying these individuals uncovered important innate immune responses, particularly the CD8+ cell non-cytotoxic antiviral response, which we believe is responsible for their control of HIV (see below).

Once we isolated ARVs, I recognized that my laboratory was not equipped to undertake the molecular approaches to clone the virus. I therefore visited Bill Rutter at UCSF who recommended that we work with his new company, Chiron Corporation. Based on my background in research at the NIH and elsewhere, I was reluctant to join with industry. That was certainly the feeling of many researchers at the time. After visiting the Chiron facility and seeing the equipment and personnel, I realized that we could clone the virus much more quickly working with the Chiron group.

We began a collaboration with Paul Luciw and Dino Dina and were successful in being the first to clone HIV (apparently by 6 days) (14). We could have reached this objective sooner if the Chiron group was not convinced by discussions with Robert Gallo that the virus resembled HTLV. Thus, they used tagged sequences from HTLV to obtain the proviral copies of ARV-2. I insisted that they use some of the proviral DNA that we were obtaining from acutely infected PBMC in our laboratory, but they felt that the HTLV probe would work. When it did not after a month, they accepted my viewpoint and within 3 weeks we had the ARV-2 clone. Subsequently, the total sequence of the virus was defined and the viral proteins identified (15).

Returning to your request for information about clinicians involved AIDS, I should say that I was the only practicing clinician who played a major role in isolating the causative virus and showing its relationship to AIDS and associated conditions. I saw the patients whom we studied in the early 1980's and cultured their PBMC. I continue to see our study subjects in my office. I perform the venipuncture, interview the subjects, and do a physical examination. There is no question that the reports from Michael Gottlieb and others suggested to the world that a new type of immune deficiency with diseases usually associated with immune disorders was occurring. Now it appears that the same kind of syndrome was probably observed in the United States and the Western countries long before (some felt in the 1950's). However, the transmission at that time was so limited that the cause of the death from opportunistic infections or cancer was not assumed to be related to a virus that attacked the immune system.

5

Raising the attention of scientists and the world to a new disease syndrome is very important, particularly one that leads to the fatal suppression of immune reponses. Therefore, the discovery of a virus that can destroy the immune system so readily as HIV does is an important and unprecedented observation. It is also noteworthy that a related lentivirus, the equine infectious anemia virus (EIAV), was probably the second virus discovered in nature (16). Thus this family of viruses was already known, and yet EIAV had not yet been identified as a lentivirus. Moreover, a D type simian retrovirus was also found in the early 1980's to be associated with an immune deficiency in monkeys at UC Davis. That finding provided support to the idea that a retrovirus could be involved in human AIDS (17).

Probably the most important impact of the discovery of HIV is the current challenge that it represents for treatment, particularly a cure, and a vaccine. Because HIV infects and becomes part of the cellular genome, the ability to eradicate the virus from the immune system and other tissues is very difficult and has not been achieved. New directions, perhaps modeled after "cures" of bacteriophages, need to be discovered such as removal of the integrated virus from the cell without killing the cell (18). The challenge of the development of a vaccine that prevents spread of a virus by infected cells as well as by the free virus also should be appreciated. This importance of the infected cell, made many years ago (19), has still not received the full attention that it merits. Immunity maintained at mucosal sites must prevent the rapid passage of HIV to the host. It is for this reason that studies of innate immune responses must be emphasized (20).

In summary, further research with discoveries that provide a means of eliminating the virus from a cell without killing the cell and preventing transmission of the virus by an infected cell will bring new paradigms for treatment and vaccines to the AIDS field and others. For example, our finding in healthy HIV-infected individuals that their CD8+ cells can suppress virus replication without killing the infected cells is a novel observation in immunology (20-22). This cytokine-mediated cellular control of viruses was previously unknown and opens up new avenues for harnessing antimicrobial responses. Since its first detection with HIV infection, this kind of CD8+ cell control virus replication has been noted for hepatitis viruses B and C as well as herpesviruses. Findings directed at the challenges of HIV infection will certainly have relevance to other medical conditions, particularly autoimmunity and cancer where control of transformed cells must be achieved.

Jay A. Levy, M.D.
University of California, San Francisco
San Francisco, CA

References

1. Gallo RC, Sarin PS, Gelmann EP, Robert-Guroff M, Richardson E, Kalyanaraman VS, Mann D, Sidhu GD, Stahl RE, Zolla-Pazner S, Leibowitch J, and Popovic M. Isolation of human T-cell leukemia virus in acquired immune deficiency syndrome (AIDS). Science, 220: 865-867 (1983).

2. Barre-Sinoussi F, Chermann J-C, Rey F, Nugeyre MT, Chamaret S, Gruest J, Dauguet C, Axler-Blin C, Vezinet-Brun F, Rouzioux C, Rozenbaum W, and Montagnier L. Isolation of a T-lymphotropic retrovirus from a patient at risk for acquired immune deficiency syndrome (AIDS). Science, 220: 868-871 (1983).

3. Hoffman AD, Banapour B, and Levy JA. Characterization of the AIDS-associated retrovirus reverse transcriptase and optimal conditions for its detection in virions. Virology, 147: 326-335 (1985).

4. Levy JA, and Henle G. Indirect immunofluorescence tests with sera from African children and cultured Burkitt's lymphoma cells. Journal of Bacteriology, 92: 275-276 (1966).

5. Kaminsky LS, McHugh T, Stites D, Volberding P, Henle G, Henle W, and Levy JA. High prevalence of antibodies to AIDS-associated retroviruses (ARV) in acquired immune deficiency syndrome and related conditions and not in other disease states. Proceedings of the National Academy of Sciences of the United States of America, 82: 5535-5539 (1985).

6. Levy JA, Mitra G, and Mozen MM. Recovery and inactivation of infectious retroviruses added to factor VIII concentrates. Lancet, ii: 722-723 (1984).

7. Popovic M, Sarngadharan MG, Read E, and Gallo RC. Detection, isolation, and continuous production of cytopathic retroviruses (HTLV-III) from patients with AIDS and pre-AIDS. Science, 224: 497-500 (1984).

8. Gallo RC, Salahuddin SZ, Popovic M, Shearer GM, Kaplan M, Haynes BF, Palker TJ, Redfield R, Oleske J, and Safai B. Frequent detection and isolation of cytopathic retroviruses (HTLV-III) from patients with AIDS and at risk for AIDS. Science, 224: 500-503 (1984).

9. Sarngadharan MG, Popovic M, Bruch L, Schupbach J, and Gallo RC. Antibodies reactive with human T-lymphotropic retroviruses (HTLV-III) in the serum of patients with AIDS. Science, 224: 506-508 (1984).

10. Schupbach J, Popovic M, Gilden RV, Gonda MA, Sangadharan MG, and Gallo RC. Serological analysis of a subgroup of human T-lymphotropic retroviruses (HTLV-III) associated with AIDS. Science, 224: 503-505 (1984).

11. Levy JA, Hoffman AD, Kramer SM, Landis JA, Shimabukuro JM, and Oshiro LS. Isolation of lymphocytopathic retroviruses from San Francisco patients with AIDS. Science, 225: 840-842 (1984).

12. Bryant ML, Yamamoto J, Luciw P, Munn R, Marx P, Higgins J, Pedersen N, Levine A, and Gardner MB. Molecular comparison of retroviruses associated with human and simian AIDS. Hematological Oncology, 3: 187-197 (1985).

13. Levy JA, Kaminsky LS, Morrow WJW, Steimer K, Luciw P, Dina D, Hoxie J, and Oshiro L. Infection by the retrovirus associated with the acquired immunodeficiency syndrome. Annals of Internal Medicine, 103: 694-699 (1985).

14. Luciw PA, Potter SJ, Steimer K, Dina D, and Levy JA. Molecular cloning of AIDS-associated retrovirus. Nature, 312: 760-763 (1984).

15. Sanchez-Pescador R, Power MD, Barr PJ, Steimer KS, Stempien MM, Brown-Shimer SL, Gee WW, Renard A, Randolph A, Levy JA, Dina D, and Luciw PA. Nucleotide sequence and expression of an AIDS-associated retrovirus (ARV-2). Science, 227: 484-492 (1985).

16. Vallee H, and Carre H. Sur l'anemie infectieuse du cheval. Comptes Rendu des Academies de Science, 139: 1239-1241 (1904).

17. Marx PA, Maul DH, Osborn KG, Lerce NW, Mordy P, Lowenstine LJ, Henrickson RV, Arthur LO, Gravell M, London WT, Sever JL, Levy JA, Munn RJ, and Gardner MB. Simian AIDS: Isolation of a type D retrovirus and disease transmission. Science, 223: 1083-1086 (1984).

18. Sarkar I, Hauber I, Hauber J, and Buchholz F. HIV-1 proviral DNA excision using an evolved recombinase. Science, 316: 1912-1915 (2007).

19. Levy JA. The transmission of AIDS: The case of the infected cell. Jama, 259: 3037-3038 (1988).

20. Levy JA. The importance of the innate immune system in controlling HIV infection and disease. Trends Immunol, 22: 312-316 (2001).

21. Walker CM, Moody DJ, Stites DP, and Levy JA. CD8+ lymphocytes can control HIV infection *in vitro* by suppressing virus replication. Science, 234: 1563-1566 (1986).

22. Levy JA. The search for the CD8+ cell anti-HIV factor (CAF). Trends in Immunol, 24: 628-632 (2003).

Endnotes

1 "Pat And Dick Get Nocturnal Welcome From Wes GOP," *The Argus*, October 5, 1956.

2 "Wesmen's Weekend First Home Game," *The Argus*, October 16, 1956.

3 "Jay Levy Conducts Frosh Vocal Group," *The Argus*, March 1, 1957.

4 "Jay Returns To Wesleyan, Stu To Williams; Twins Reveal Complete Identity Hoax Story," *The Argus*, February 18, 1958.

5 "CB Candidates Open Campaign By Endorsing Varying Reforms," *The Argus*, February 20, 1959.

6 "Letter To The Editor," *The Argus*, March 3, 1959.

7 "Levy Cops Vice Presidency; Hogendorn Is Sec. – Treasurer," *The Argus*, March 5, 1959.

8 "Campus Fraternities Pledge Record Low Of 160," *The Argus*, September 19, 1958.

9 "These Girls Will Attend Fall House Party Weekend," *The Argus*, November 15, 1957.

10 "The Highwaymen Biography," Allmusic.com.

11 "The Argus Uncovers History Of Progressive Frat's Rebellion," *The Argus*, November 21, 2013.

12 "Crow Chapter Cites Background of Suspension," *The Argus*, October 17, 1958.

13 "Crow Members Suspended By National Rule Last Night," *The Argus*, October 10, 1958.

14 "Crow's Alumni To Be Briefed By Mayo On Ritual Revision," *The Argus*, June 5, 1959.

15 "Students' Votes Favor Nixon, But Faculty Strong For Jack," *The Argus*, November 4, 1960.

16 "Senate Passes Motion To End Subfrosh Deals," *The Argus*, April 21, 1959.

17 "From Yellow Berets to Nobel Laureates: The Vietnam War and NIH's Clinical Associates Program," *The NIH Catalyst*, March-April 2021.

18 "The AIDS Epidemic in San Francisco: The Medical Response, 1981-1984," Interview with Jay A. Levy, MD, *The San Francisco AIDS Oral History Series*, 1993.

19 J. A. Levy, T. Pincus, "Demonstration of biological activity of a murine leukemia virus in New Zealand Black mice," *Science* 1970, 170:326-327.

20 Yuan Chang, et al., "Identification of herpesvirus-like DNA sequences in AIDS-associated Kaposi's sarcoma," *Science.* (1994) Dec 16;266(5192):1865-9.

21 Jay A. Levy, *HIV and the Pathogenesis of AIDS* (ASM Press, 1994).

22 "The HIV/AIDS Epidemic in the United States: The Basics," KFF, October 9, 2024.

23 "Global HIV & AIDS statistics — Fact sheet," July 10, 2025, UNAIDS.

24 Kevin M De Cock, et al., "Reflections on 30 years of AIDS," *Emerg Infectious Disease* (2011) Jun;17(6):1044-8.

25 Anthony Fauci, MD, and H. Clifford Lane, MD, "Four Decades of AIDS – Much Accomplished, Much to Do," *The New England Journal of Medicine*, July 2, 2020.

26 Luc Montagnier, "Biographical," The Nobel Prize, 2008.

27 "*Pneumocystis* Pneumonia – Los Angeles," *Morbidity and Mortality Weekly Report*, June 5, 1981.

28 "New Homosexual Disorder Worries Health Officials," *The New York Times*, May 11, 1982.

29 "HIV & AIDS," Cleveland Clinic, June 6, 2022.

30 Jay A. Levy, "The Importance of Basic Science in HIV/AIDS and Future Pandemics," *Memory Lives On: Documenting the HIV/AIDS Epidemic*, April 1, 2021.

31 Randy Shilts, "UC Assailed for Delay on AIDS Funds," *San Francisco Chronicle*, August 25, 1983.

32 Levy, *Memory Lives On.*

33 Randy Shilts, *And the Band Played On: Politics, People, and the AIDS Epidemic* (St. Martin's Press, 1987), xxiii.

34 Chang, "Identification of herpesvirus-like DNA sequences in AIDS-associated Kaposi's sarcoma," 1865-9.

35 Levy, *Memory Lives On.*

36 Jay A. Levy and John L. Ziegler, "Acquired immunodeficiency syndrome is an opportunistic infection and Kaposi's sarcoma results from secondary immune stimulation," *Lancet.* (1983) Jul 9;2(8341):78-81.

37 Françoise Barré-Sinoussi, et al., "Isolation of a T-lymphotropic retrovirus from a patient at risk for acquired immune deficiency syndrome (AIDS),"

Science. (1983) May 20;220(4599):868-71.

38 Jay A. Levy, et al., "Isolation of Lymphocytopathic Retroviruses from San Francisco Patients with AIDS," *Science* (1984) 225,840-842.

39 "AIDS Papers Heard 'Round the World," *Science*, May 5, 1997.

40 M. L. Bryant, et al., "Molecular comparison of retroviruses associated with human and simian AIDS," *Hematological Oncoloy* (1985): Jul-Sep;3(3):187-97.

41 Levy, *Memory Lives On.*

42 Ibid.

43 Robert C. Gallo, "HIV and the Pathogenesis of AIDS," *Trends in Microbiology*, Volume 3, Issue 7, 1995, 285-286.

44 Gilbert C. White, "Hemophilia: an amazing 35-year journey from the depths of HIV to the threshold of cure," *Transactions of the American Clinical and Climatological Association* (2010):121:61-73; discussion 74-5.

45 Jay A Levy, et al., "Recovery and inactivation of infectious retroviruses from factor VIII concentration," *Lancet* (1984): Sep 29;2(8405):722-3.

46 "Update: Acquired Immunodeficiency Syndrome (AIDS) in Persons with Hemophilia," *Morbidity and Mortality Weekly Report*, October 26, 1984.

47 B. L Evatt, "The tragic history of AIDS in the hemophilia population, 1982-1984," *Journal of Thrombosis and Haemostasis* (2006) Nov;4(11):2295-301.

48 Jay A. Levy, et al., "Inactivation by wet and dry heat of AIDS-associated retroviruses during factor VIII purification from plasma," *Lancet* (1985) Jun 22;1(8443):1456-7.

49 Institute of Medicine (US) Committee to Study HIV Transmission Through Blood and Blood Products; Leveton LB, Sox HC Jr., Stoto MA, editors. *HIV And The Blood Supply: An Analysis Of Crisis Decisionmaking.* Washington (DC): National Academies Press (US); 1995.

50 "The AIDS Epidemic in San Francisco: The Medical Response, 1981-1984," Interview with Jay A. Levy, MD, *The San Francisco AIDS Oral History Series*, 1993.

51 "The Unbeliever," *The New York Times*, April 7, 1996.

52 Jon Cohen, "The Duesberg phenomenon," *Science* (1994) Dec 9; 266(5191): 1642-4.

53 "Global HIV & AIDS statistics — Fact sheet," July 10, 2025, UNAIDS.

54 "HIV/AIDS," Our World in Data, December 2023.

55 Alan L. Landay, et al., "Chronic fatigue syndrome: clinical condition associated with immune activation," *Lancet* (1991): Sep 21;338(8769):707-12.

56 "Anasse '18 Reflects on Impact of UCSF Science Camp," *The Wesleyan Connection*, October 20, 2017.

57 "Drug-Resistant Superbugs: CIMAR Symposium Examines the Intersection of People, Animals, Food, and the Environment, and Their Impact on Health," Stuart B. Levy Center for Integrated Management of Antimicrobial Resistance, April 9, 2019.

58 Stuart B. Levy, et al., "Changes in intestinal flora of farm personnel after introduction of a tetracycline-supplemented feed on a farm," *The New England Journal of Medicine* (1976) Sep 9;295(11):583-8.

59 "Stuart Levy Changed Science, Public Policy on Antibiotics," *The Wall Street Journal*, September 27, 2019.

60 "Stuart B Levy," *Lancet*, October 12, 2019.

61 "Remembering Stuart Levy," TuftsNow, September 13, 2019.

62 "The Antibiotic Paradox: How the Misuse of Antibiotics Destroys Their Curative Powers," *The New England Journal of Medicine*, October 10, 2002.

63 *Frontiers in Antimicrobial Resistance: A Tribute to Stuart B. Levy* (American Society for Microbiology, 2005).

64 "Stuart Levy, microbiologist who sounded alarm on antibiotic resistance, dies at 80," *The Washington Post*, September 19, 2019.

65 "Remembering Stuart Levy," TuftsNow, September 13, 2019.

66 "Stuart B. Levy, M.D. (November 21, 1938 – September 4, 2019): A Trailblazing Force in the Fight Against Antimicrobial Resistance," Stuart B. Levy Center for Integrated Management of Antimicrobial Resistance.

67 R. Ellen Koenig, et al., "HIV Infection in the Dominican Republic-Reply," *JAMA* (1987): 258(1):47.

68 "Jeannette Tenthorey, PhD, named the inagural Jay A. Levy Endowed Professor in Virology in September, 2025," UC San Francisco.

69 "Understanding Immunity: Jeannette Tenthorey," Howard Hughes Medical Institute, December 12, 2024.

70 "Pioneering HIV Researcher Donates 'Important' Career Collection to UCSF," UC San Francisco, January 21, 2025.